Welcome to Ātman Magazine.

In this issue:

# HINDU GODDESSES

## Temples of Gokulum, Mysore India

## BUY THE TICKET, *Take the Ride*

## Ashtanga Secondary Series

## Opening & Closing Chants
(and a few more for good measure.)

# DURGA

The tale of Durga and her battle against the demons is a captivating legend from Hindu mythology, symbolizing the triumph of good over evil. According to the myth, there was a demon king named Mahishasura who had performed intense penance to obtain a boon from Lord Brahma, granting him invincibility against all male beings. Empowered by this boon, Mahishasura wreaked havoc across the three worlds, threatening the balance of cosmic order.
As the situation grew dire, the gods in heaven sought a solution to defeat Mahishasura. They combined their divine energies, and from their collective power emerged the radiant goddess Durga. Adorned with celestial weapons and riding atop a fierce lion, Durga epitomized courage, strength, and divine grace. She was the embodiment of Shakti, the divine feminine energy.
The battle between Durga and Mahishasura raged on for nine days and nights, culminating in a fierce confrontation. With her unparalleled prowess, Durga vanquished the demon king, piercing him with her trident and bringing an end to his reign of terror. The victory of Durga symbolizes the eternal struggle between good and evil, reaffirming the belief that righteousness will always prevail over darkness.
Durga's triumph is celebrated annually during the festival of Navaratri, where devotees honor her divine presence and seek her blessings for protection and prosperity. Her story serves as a powerful reminder of the indomitable spirit within each individual to overcome challenges and adversities with courage, determination, and faith.

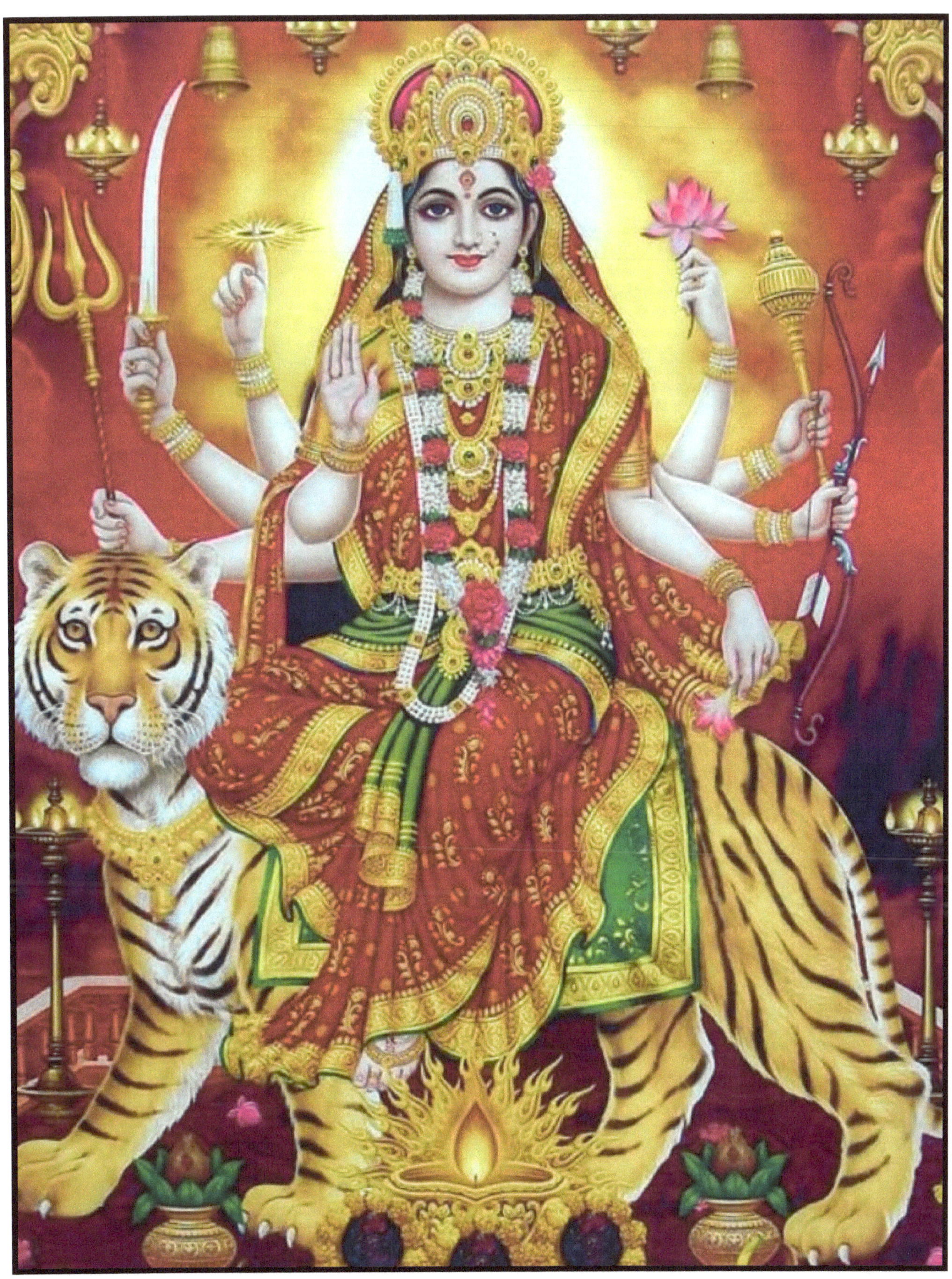

# SARASWATI

Saraswati is the goddess of knowledge, music, arts, wisdom, and learning. Her story is deeply intertwined with the fabric of Hindu cosmology and mythology.

According to the Hindu scriptures, Saraswati is said to have emerged during the creation of the universe. In the Rigveda, one of the oldest texts in Hinduism, she is revered as a river goddess. She is described as a beautiful deity adorned with white garments, symbolizing purity and knowledge.

The legend of Saraswati's origin varies across different texts and traditions, but a commonly cited myth is her emergence during the cosmic creation known as "Saraswati Sukta." According to this legend, when Lord Brahma, the creator of the universe, set about the task of creation, he realized that he needed a companion who could help him bring order to the chaos. As he meditated upon this, a divine being manifested from his mouth. This celestial being was Saraswati, radiant and graceful, embodying the essence of knowledge and creativity.

As the consort of Brahma, Saraswati represents the feminine aspect of creation. Together, they symbolize the union of intellect and creativity, essential for the process of creation and sustenance in the universe.

Saraswati is often depicted sitting on a lotus flower, symbolizing purity, with a Veena (a stringed musical instrument) in her hands, representing the arts and creativity.

Saraswati is revered not only as the goddess of learning but also as the source of inspiration for poets, musicians, scholars, and artists. She is worshipped by students seeking wisdom and knowledge, as well as by those engaged in creative pursuits. Her blessings are sought before undertaking any new venture, whether it be the beginning of a new academic year, the inauguration of a new business, or the commencement of an artistic endeavor.

In Hindu mythology, Saraswati's significance extends beyond her role as a goddess. She embodies the eternal quest for knowledge and enlightenment, inspiring devotees to seek truth and wisdom. Her presence is believed to reside in the flow of rivers, the melody of music, the rhythm of poetry, and the depths of scholarly pursuits, reminding humanity of the sacred connection between knowledge, creativity, and spirituality.

of body text

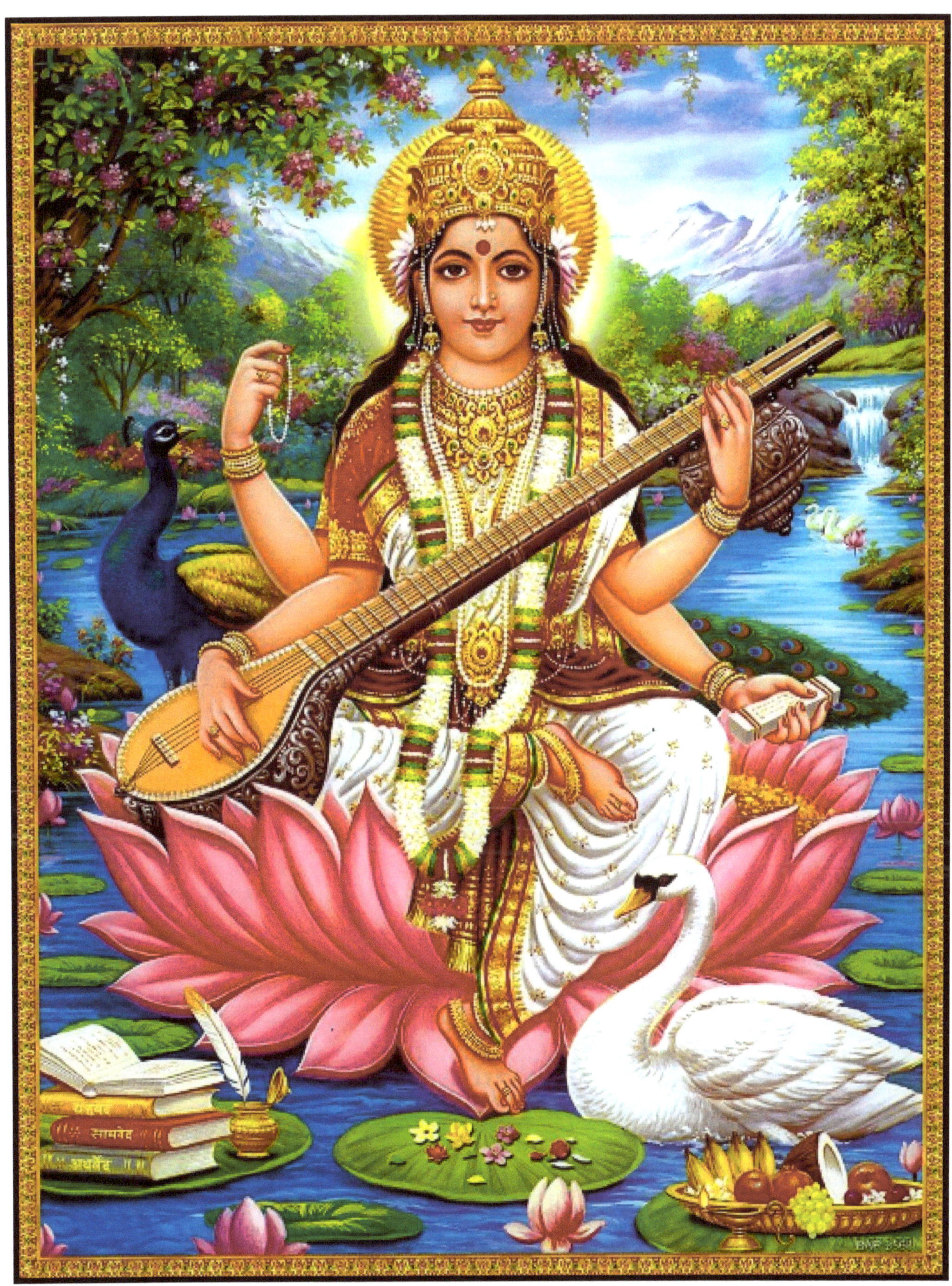

# LAKSHMI

Lakshmi, the goddess of wealth, prosperity, and fortune, has a captivating story in Hindu mythology. Her origin is closely associated with the churning of the cosmic ocean, a legendary event known as the Samudra Manthan.

According to the ancient texts, the Devas (celestial beings) and the Asuras (demons) once decided to collaborate to churn the ocean of milk in order to obtain the nectar of immortality, known as Amrita. However, they needed a central support to churn the ocean, and Mount Mandara served that purpose, acting as the churning rod.

During the churning, numerous divine beings and treasures emerged from the ocean. One of the most significant beings to emerge was Lakshmi, radiantly beautiful and adorned with divine attributes. She arose from the ocean seated on a lotus, symbolizing purity and transcendence.

As Lakshmi emerged, she captivated everyone with her grace and charm. The Devas, recognizing her divine nature and the auspiciousness she represented, welcomed her with reverence. They recognized her as the embodiment of abundance, prosperity, and auspiciousness.

In Hindu mythology, Lakshmi is often depicted as the consort of Lord Vishnu, the preserver of the universe. Their union symbolizes the harmonious balance between wealth and righteousness. Lakshmi's presence brings prosperity and abundance into the lives of devotees, while Vishnu's guidance ensures that wealth is used for the benefit of all beings and for upholding righteousness.

Lakshmi's blessings are sought by devotees for material wealth, spiritual prosperity, and overall well-being. She is worshipped fervently during festivals such as Diwali, the festival of lights, where devotees illuminate their homes to welcome her and seek her blessings for a prosperous year ahead.

Lakshmi's story serves as a reminder of the importance of wealth and abundance in life, but also emphasizes the need for humility, righteousness, and the ethical use of resources. She teaches that true prosperity lies not only in material wealth but also in spiritual richness and the well-being of all beings in the universe.

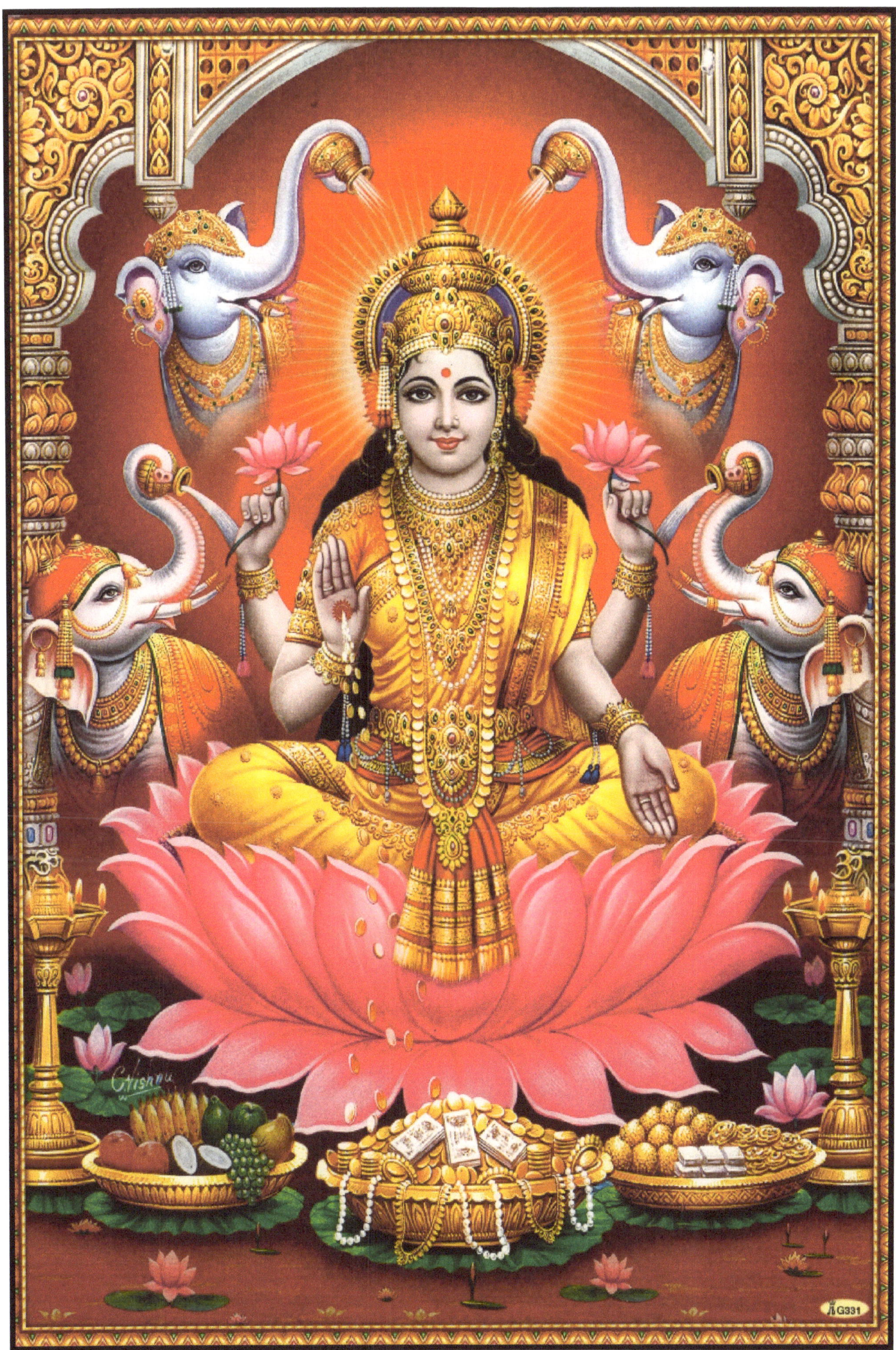

# KALI

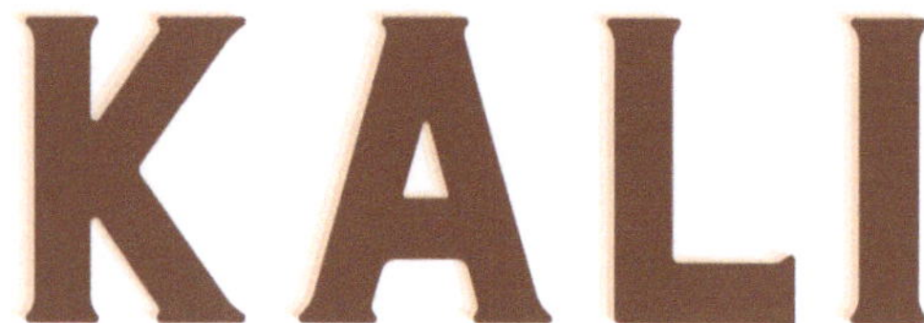

Kali emerged during a cosmic battle between the Devas (celestial beings) and the Asuras (demons). The demon Raktabija had a unique power: whenever a drop of his blood fell on the ground, a clone of him would manifest, making him nearly invincible. The Devas, unable to defeat Raktabija, turned to the divine feminine for help.

In response to their prayers, Kali emerged from the forehead of the goddess Durga, a fierce and powerful form of the divine mother. Kali's appearance was striking and terrifying. She was adorned with a garland of skulls, her tongue protruded out, and she wielded various weapons in her multiple hands. Her appearance symbolized the destruction of ego and the eradication of ignorance.

When Kali entered the battlefield, she unleashed her wrath upon Raktabija and his clones. With her ferocious demeanor and unstoppable force, she vanquished the demon and put an end to his reign of terror. She drank his blood before it could touch the ground, thereby preventing the creation of new clones. In this act, Kali demonstrated her role as the destroyer of evil forces and the protector of cosmic order.

However, Kali's story goes beyond her role as a fierce warrior goddess. She also embodies the transformative power of time and the cycles of creation and destruction in the universe. Kali is often depicted dancing amidst the flames of destruction, representing the eternal dance of life and death.

In Hindu tradition, Kali is worshipped as the divine mother who grants liberation and spiritual awakening to her devotees. Despite her fearsome appearance, she is believed to be compassionate towards those who seek her guidance with sincerity and devotion.

Kali's story serves as a reminder of the cyclical nature of existence, where destruction paves the way for new beginnings and transformation. She teaches that by confronting our fears and embracing change, we can attain liberation from the bonds of ignorance and ego, ultimately leading to spiritual enlightenment.

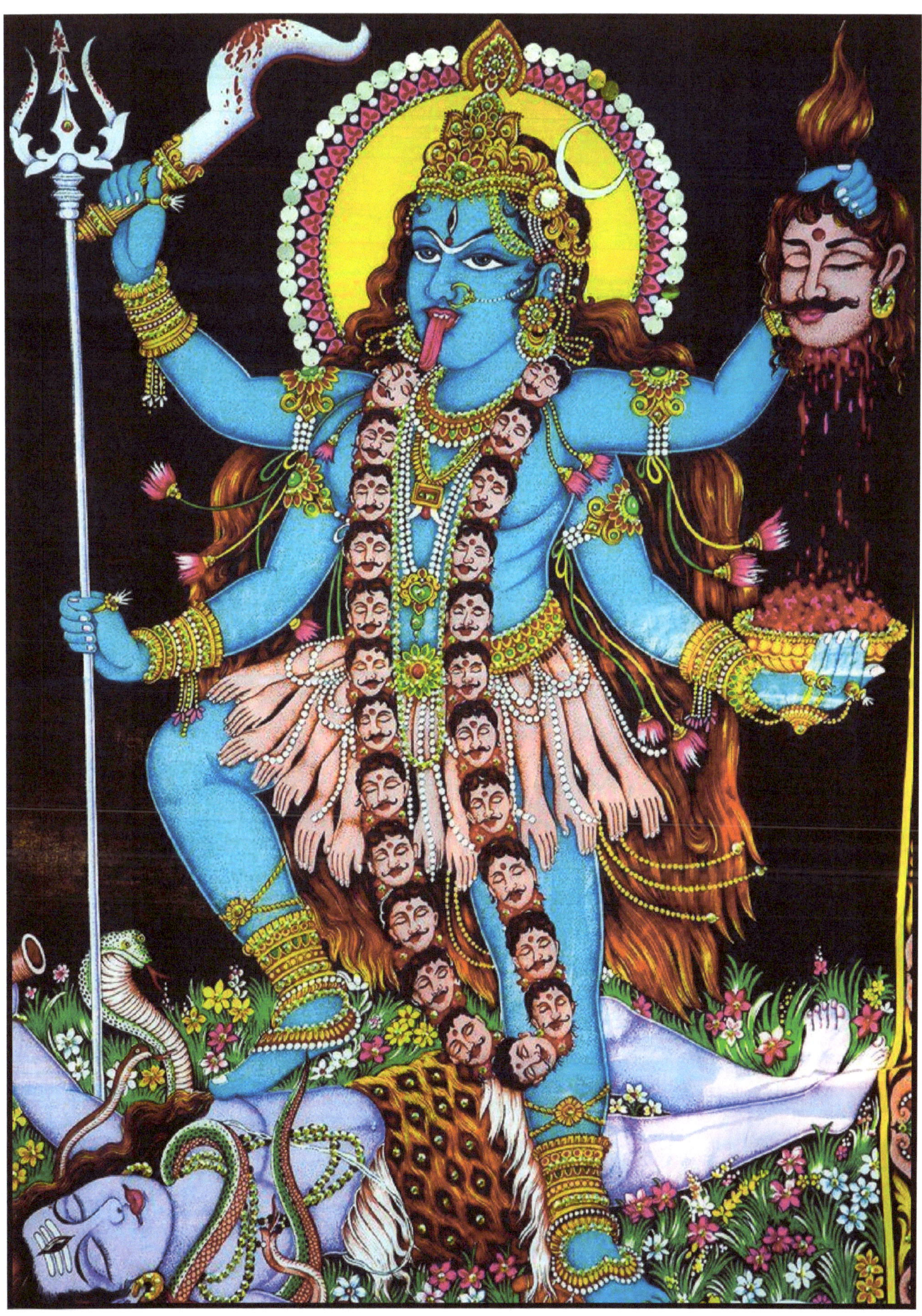

# PARVATI

Parvati, is one of the most beloved goddesses in Hindu mythology. She is revered as the divine mother, representing love, fertility, and devotion. Parvati's story is rich with symbolism and reflects the deep philosophical concepts of Hinduism. Parvati is the daughter of King Himavan, the personification of the Himalayan mountains, and Queen Mainavati. From a young age, Parvati was drawn to Lord Shiva, the ascetic god of destruction and transformation. She was captivated by his meditative presence and sought to win his affection through her devotion and penance.

Legend has it that Pavati undertook severe austerities and penances to please Lord Shiva and win his hand in marriage. She immersed herself in rigorous practices, enduring harsh conditions and extreme hardships. Her unwavering dedication and purity of heart caught the attention of Shiva, who was deeply moved by her devotion.

Impressed by Parvati's commitment, Shiva eventually agreed to marry her, recognizing her as his divine counterpart, Shakti. Their union symbolized the harmonious balance between the masculine and feminine energies in the universe. Parvati, as the consort of Shiva, became known as Parvati, a name derived from the word "parvat," meaning mountain, reflecting her divine lineage.

Parvati's marriage to Shiva is celebrated as a sacred union, embodying the ideals of love, devotion, and spiritual partnership. Together, they represent the divine aspects of creation, preservation, and destruction, essential for the perpetuation of the cosmic cycle.

As the divine mother, Parvati is worshipped in various forms and manifestations across Hindu tradition. She is revered as Durga, the fierce warrior goddess who vanquishes evil forces, and as Kali, the formidable goddess of time and transformation. Parvati is also celebrated as Annapurna, the goddess of nourishment, and Gauri, the epitome of marital bliss and harmony.

Parvati's story serves as an inspiration for devotees, highlighting the power of love, devotion, and perseverance in the pursuit of spiritual fulfillment. Her unwavering dedication to Lord Shiva symbolizes the soul's quest for union with the divine, transcending the dualities of the material world to attain spiritual enlightenment.

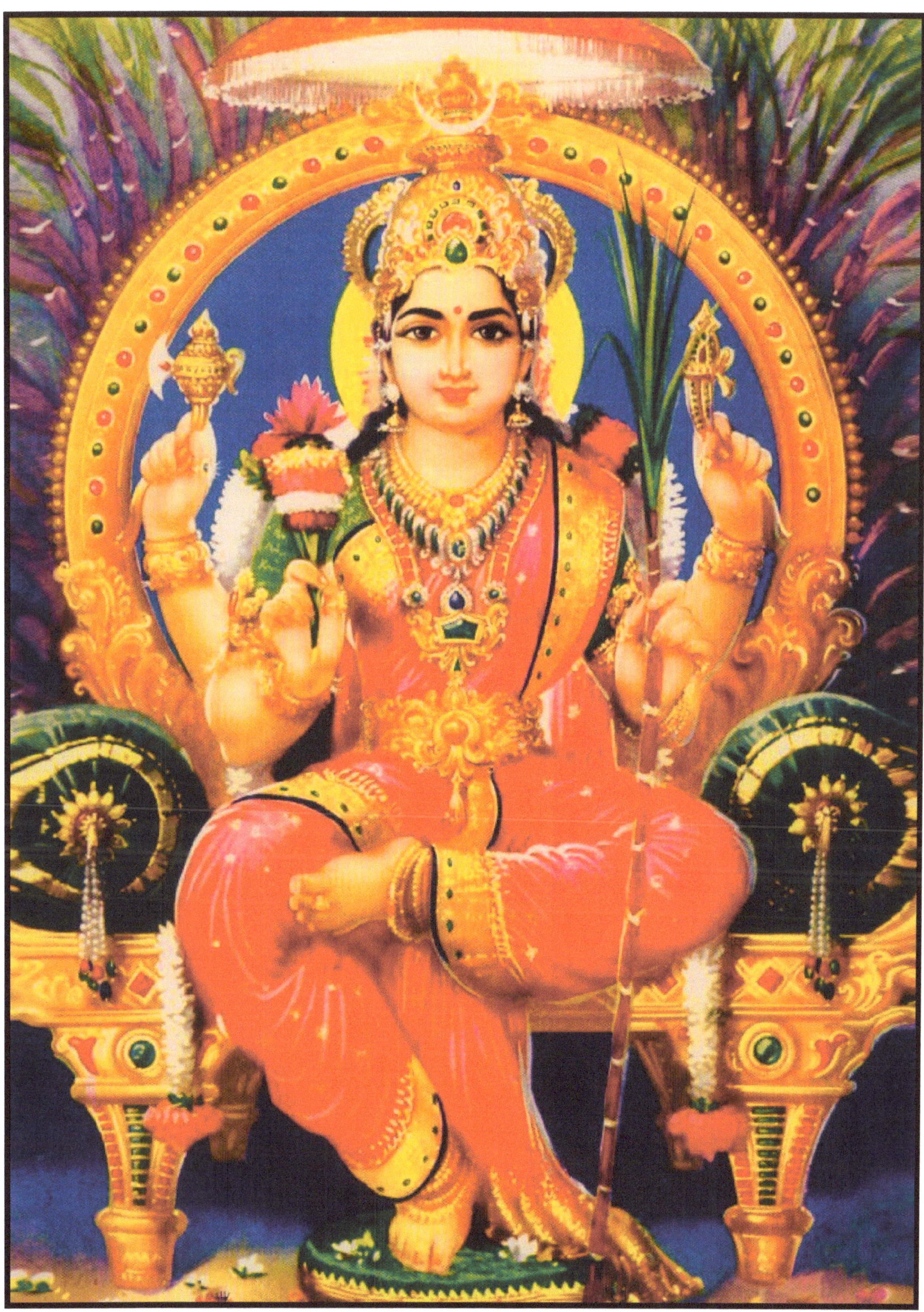

# ARDHANARISHVARA

Ardhanarishvara is a combination of three words 'Ardha', 'Nari' and 'Ishwara' means 'half', 'woman' and 'lord' respectively, which when combined means the lord whose half is woman. It is believed that the God is Lord Shiva and the woman part is his consort Goddess Parvati or Shakti. The Ardhanarishvara represents a constructive and generative power. There is a legend about the Ardhanarishvara form of god.

## Legend of Ardhanarishvara

Sage Bringi was one of the ardent followers of Lord Shiva. He used to worship only Lord Shiva but not Shakti. Goddess Shakti, being the power of the universe pulled out the energy from Bringi Maharishi's body. Now he was even unable to stand. The sage then pleaded to god. God Shiva provided him with a stick.

The Rishi could walk with the support of the stick and continued worshipping Lord Shiva alone. Goddess Shakti wanted to become an inseparable part of Lord Shiva. She started observing Kedara Mahavrata austerity, which is also known as Deepavali. Lord Shiva was propitiated with the austerity and granted her boon of being part to his own form. The Lord thus became Ardhanarishvara.

This is one of the very important forms of the god worshipped by Hindus. The reference of Ardhanarishvara is found in many Hindu scriptures. God is beyond the concept of any sex. So God can be male, female, and even neuter too. So god exists in intrinsic condition as is referred by Ardhanarishvara.

Philosophically this form is quite associated with the grace of God. The formless god is called Parashiva. The god creates the world and act for the benefits of Pashus (souls), who are attached by Pasha (bondage). The power of creation comes from Shiva and Shakti. Though they are incorporated in the same form they act independently as well as jointly. This is understood when the philosophers in ancient scriptures describe Shakti as wife, mother and daughter of Shiva. As wife, Shakti acts together with Shiva, as mother Shakti becomes Shiva or Shiva comes out of Shakti and as daughter Shiva becomes Shakti.

India from its ancient time has many sculptures and paintings of Ardhanarishvara, which are found in various poses, like 'Abhanga', a posture with only one curve, 'Tribhanga', a posture with mild three curves and 'Atibhanga', a posture with extreme curves. Thus maleness and femaleness are contained in one frame in Ardhanarishvara.

## Symbolism of Ardhanarishvara

Ardhanarishvara symbolizes male and female principles cannot be separated. It conveys the unity of opposites in the universe. The male half stands for Purusha and female half is Prakriti. The union of Purusha (Shiva) and Prakriti (Shiva's energy, Shakti) generates the universe. Mahabharata lauds this form as the source of creation. Ardhanarishvara harmonizes the two conflicting ways of life: the spiritual way of the ascetic as represented by Shiva, and the materialistic way of the householder symbolized by Parvati. It conveys that Shiva and Shakti are one and the same.

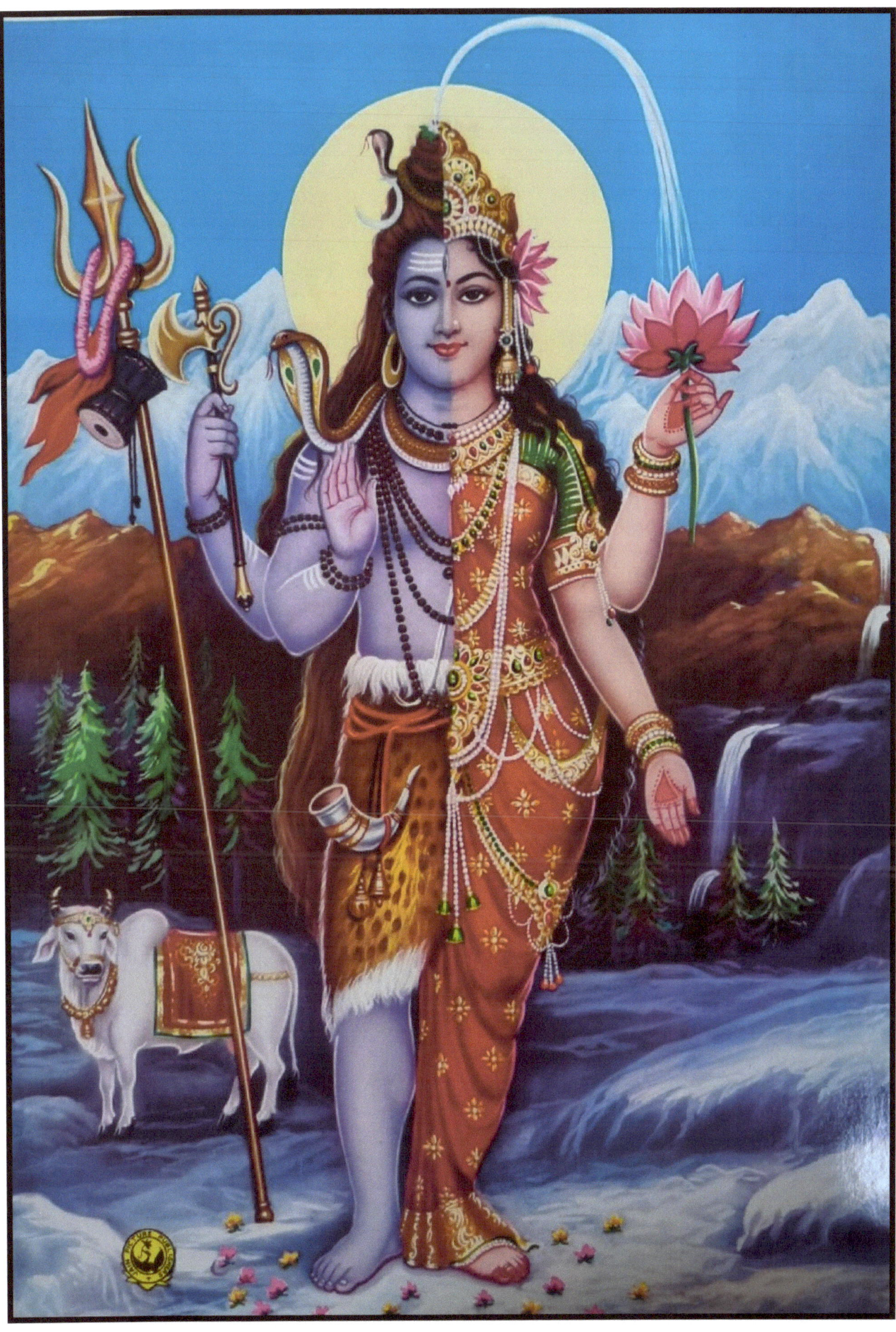

# BUY THE TICKET, *Take the Ride*

So you've been practicing for a whaile and you're thinkibg about going to inida. Just buy the ticket, and take the ride!  Here are some steps to get you practicing at "the source" of ashtnga yoga.

1. Research Yoga Schools: There are a few to choose from.  The most obvious is the Sharath [Jois] Yoga Center.  It can be tricky to secure your spot, but once done, you made it to the big leagues. You can also go with the tried and true, KPJAYI run by Saraswati Jois, daughter of P. Jois and mother of S. Jois).  She has smaller crowds and is in Gokulum so a long commute isn't necessary.  There is also Ashtanga Saadhana ran by Vijay Kumar. A teacher that can stand on his own merit.

2. Check Visa Requirements: If you are coming from the USA, you will need a VISA.  You can get an e-visa in the course of a few days.  It a simole process, but read the fine print.  It's of this author's option to NOT claim you are entering the country to do any thing yoga related as they my suspect that you are trying to make moeny and will demand a work VISA.

3. Book Accommodation: There are plenty of places to stay within walking distance of KPJAYI, and that's where must people stay.  Renting a single or double room is as easy as googling  "rooms to rent in Mysore".  It will run you about $250-$500 in peak season but cheaper in the low season. Most apartments rent by the full month, so if you are coming half way through the month be prepared to negotiate a price that's fair for you.

4. Plan Your Budget: Calculate the cost of tuition, accommodation, food, transportation, and any additional expenses like travel insurance and excursions. Also think about the money you will NOT be making when you're gone.  Many a yogi returns home broke and stay broke because they didn't think far enough ahead.

5. Arrange Travel: Book your flights to Bengaluru International Airport, the nearest major airport to Mysore, and plan your transportation from the airport to Mysore. Easiest way is to take the "Flybus".

6. Obtain Necessary Vaccinations: Check with your doctor or a travel clinic to see if any vaccinations are recommended or required for travel to India.  Most likely not, but you never know.  Google the nearest western hosiptal and put it in your "saved" google maps file.

7. Pack Essentials: Prepare your yoga attire, comfortable clothing, toiletries, any necessary medications, and any items specific to your stay in India. You'll be able to pick up anything you left behind in stores there.  Have some fun and head to the store for toothpaste only to pick up hand cream by mistake.

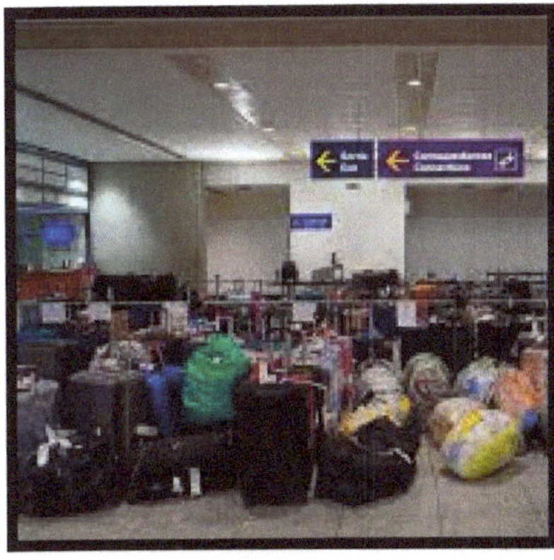


8. **Prepare for the Climate:** Mysore can be hot and humid, so pack lightweight and breathable clothing, as well as sun protection like sunscreen and a hat. No need to buy travel clothes, just pack what's already in your closet, or less. Shirts, pants, skirts and rugs are  great souvenirs to bring home.

9. **Learn Basic Phrases:** Familiarize yourself with basic phrases in Kannada, the local language, to help you navigate and communicate more easily. You can always use google translate, but a warm "hello", "good morning" and/or "thank you." goes a long way.

10. **Plan Your Itinerary:** Research local attractions and activities to enjoy during your free time, such as exploring Mysore Palace, visiting local markets, or taking day trips to nearby sights.  After practice the whole day awaits you!  Don't fly half way around the world, only to get to know the walls of your apartment, EXPLORE, GET LOST, HAVE FUN!

11. **Stay Open-Minded:** Approach your yoga studies with an open mind and a willingness to learn from different teachers and experiences.  Go to a chanting class, learn how to cook, rent a scooter, so many things to do.

12. **Enjoy Your Journey:** Embrace the unique culture and atmosphere of Mysore, immerse yourself in your yoga practice, and savor every moment of your transformative journey. Document it.  Yes, be that annoying tourist who takes pictures of EVERYTHING!  You'll have plenty to photograph.

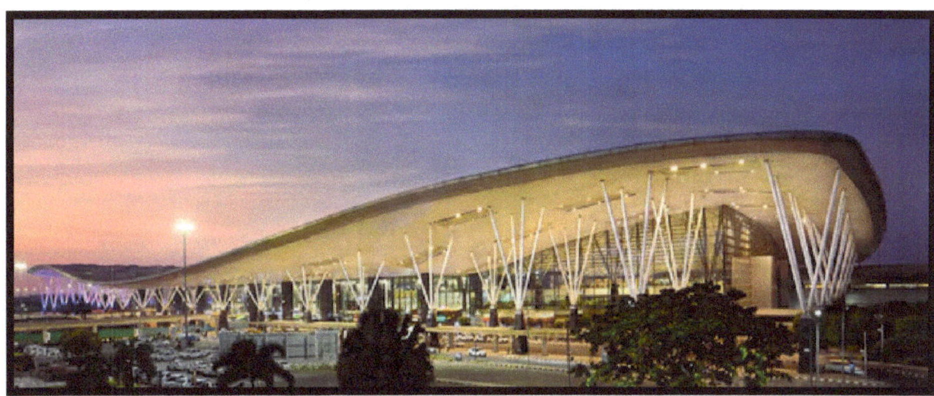

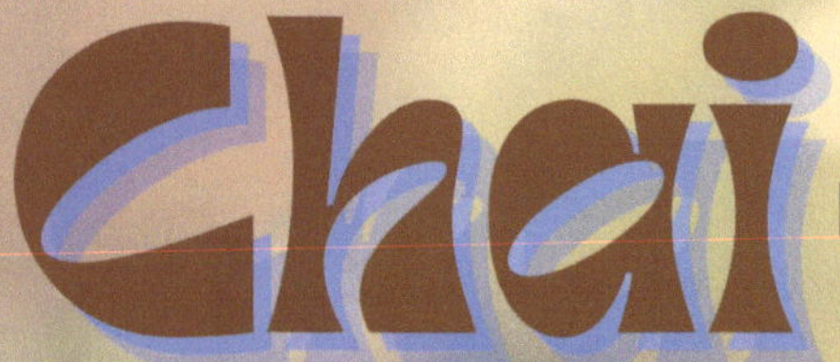

# Chai

**by Lakshmi Sriram / @laksri1999**

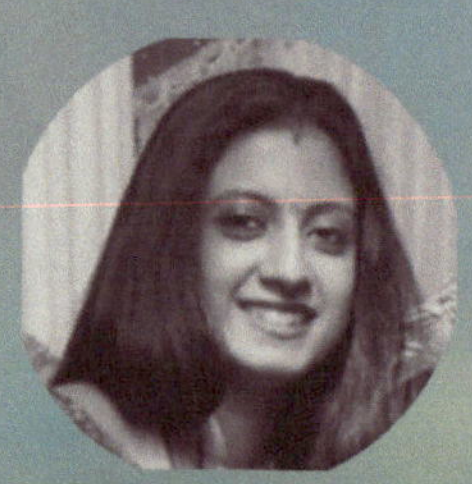

Chances are , if you are addicted to caffeine then at some point alongwith coffee you would have had tea as well. Tea also known as chai , is the most popular beverage had by practically every Indian , right from your daily wage worker, to people working in every sector from the lowest to the highest rank. A chai break is always the trend for any tea lover, be it at the early dawn when they start the day or at mid morning/afternoon, evening and night as well.

What is Chai? It's a beverage made out of milk, sugar and tea leaves. There is the masala chai or spiced tea, as well that's made using spices like cardamom, cinnamon, fennel, ginger, pepper and some more. Chai originates in India where ancient royals drank a healing beverage made with different spices and milk. The early name for masala chai was kadha , and considered a magical drink for curing communicable illnesses like sore throat, cold, cough, headache and fever.

Legend states that Masala chai's foundations were laid some 5000 years ago when Indian emperors used to sip a brewed concoction of spices to remain alert throughout courtly affairs . The drink was caffeine free and used as an ayurvedic medicine. It wasn't until 1835 and the British intervention when Black tea leaves were introduced.

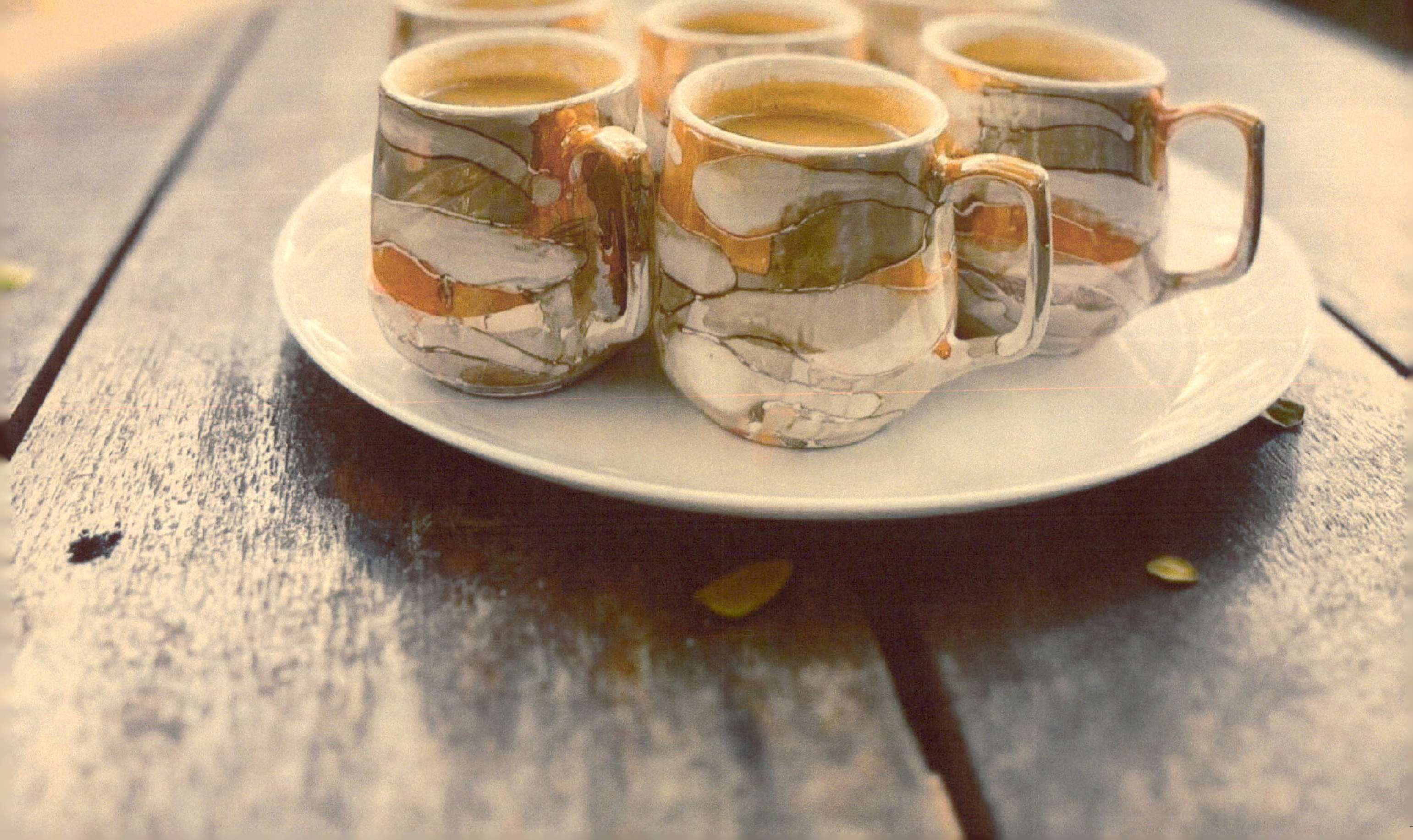

The British gave tea out for free in the beginning. They convinced lobbies to give Indian workers a tea break in which they could consume tea. They even put up signs in different Indian languages to teach people how to brew tea. Tea shops were set up at the newly built railway stations which helped tea spread throughout India. As black tea was the most expensive ingredient, vendors used milk, sugar and spices to keep their brews flavorful while holding costs down. Masal Chai's popularity spread.

Regionally, street vendors and train vendors called chai wallahs (" tea persons ", kind of like a barista of Chai) serve masala chai to the public. Chai is also used to welcome guests into the home.

In some areas, people drink an average of four small cups of Chai per day. A popular time for chai is around 4 pm with an afternoon snack. This snack may include savory treats like Samosas, pakoras, farsan (Gujarati snacks) and nashta,( savory breakfast foods that double as snack foods).

To brew chai , the first step is to simmer the spices in a saucepan with a cup or so of water. Then, once the flavours have blended and infused, add black tea and let it brew as you normally brew it. Experimentation is the key to learning how to create your own perfect spice mix and tea ratio. You can make it as strong and spicy as you like it. After a few minutes of the brewing, strain the spices and coarse tea out. Finally add milk , as little or as much as you like, to make everything rich and creamy. You can add any milk but whole cow's milk is best as its high fat content balances well with the spice mix. Full cream or sweetened condensed milk also work well. While the flavors may be complex, the process is not.

When are you going to make yourself a cup of Chai then??

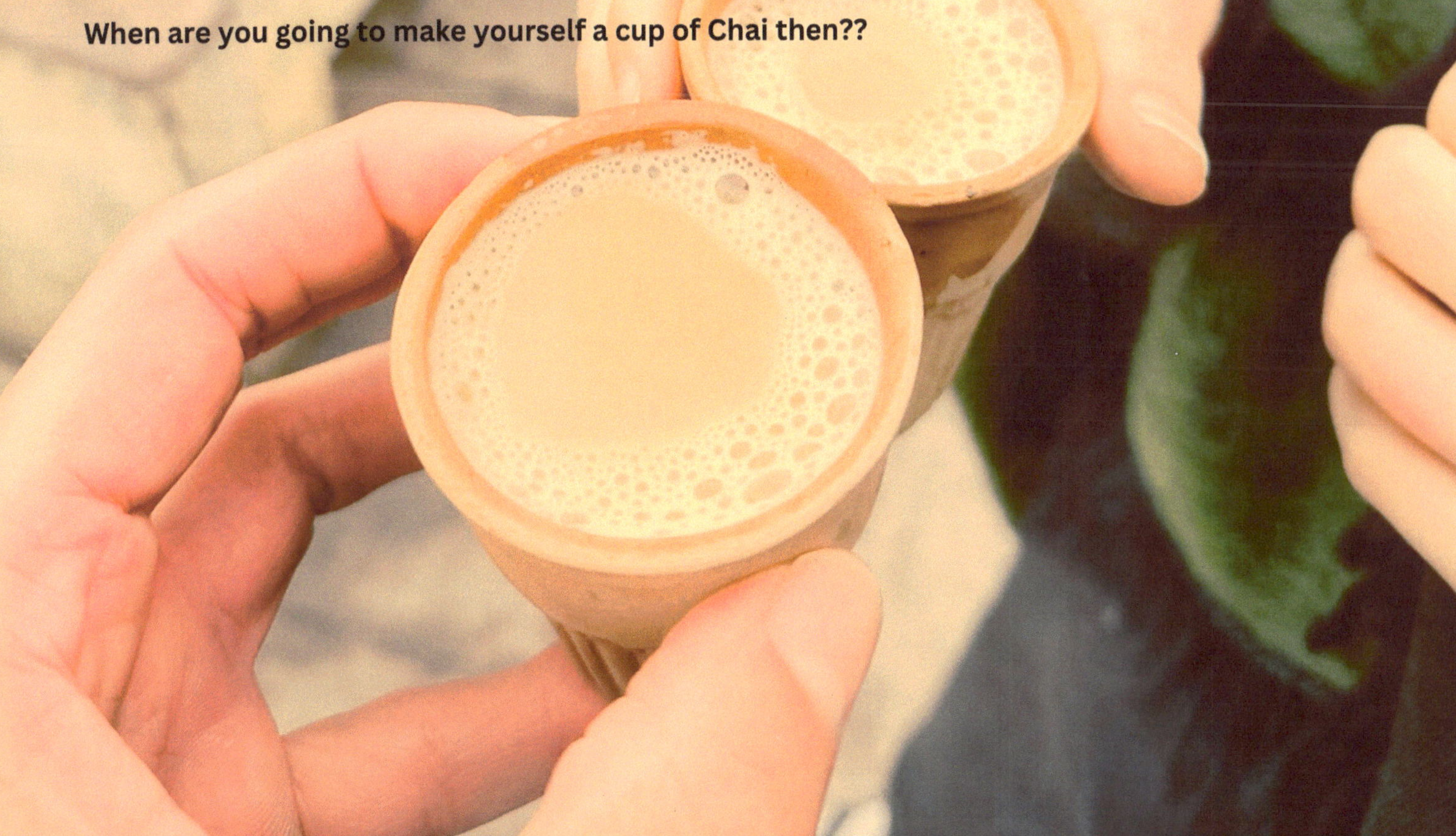

# ASHTANGA YOGA Second Series

ashtangayogaross.com

## Sūryanamaskāra A

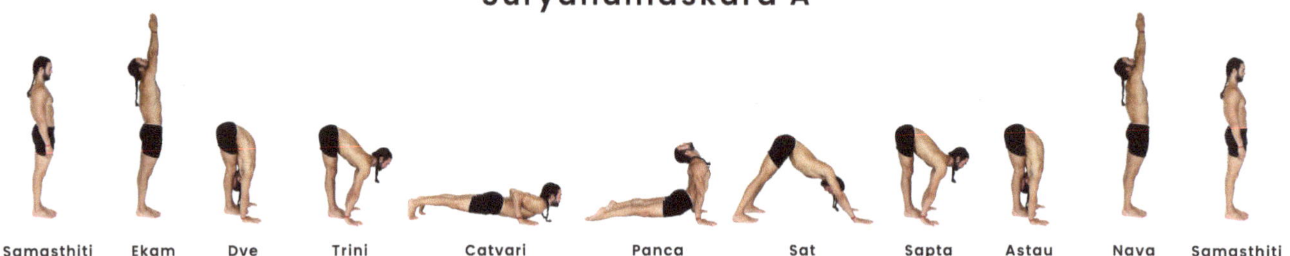

Samasthiti   Ekam   Dve   Trini   Catvari   Panca   Sat   Sapta   Astau   Nava   Samasthiti

## Sūryanamaskāra B

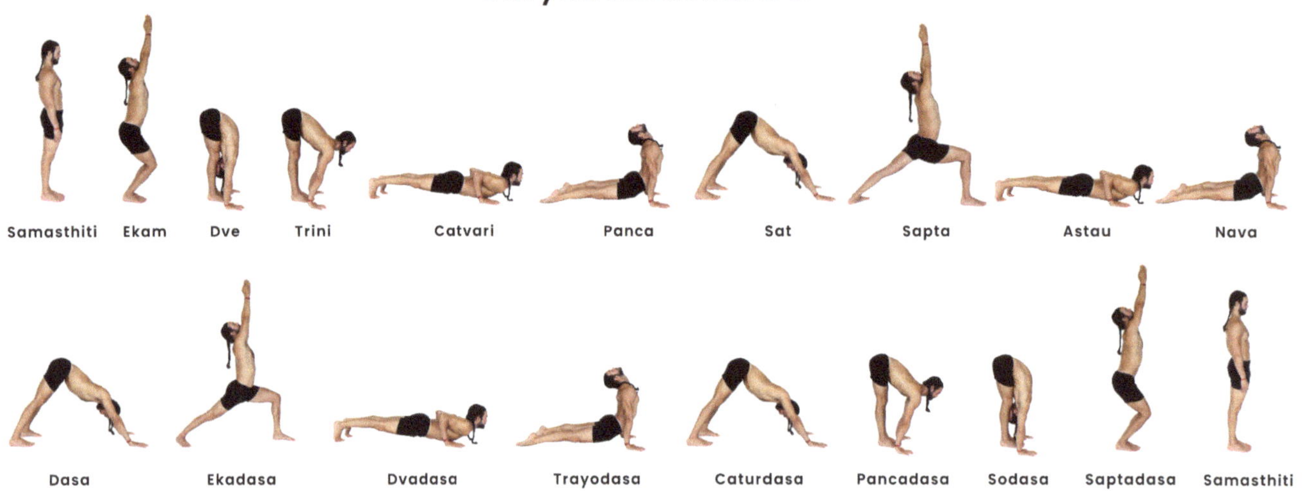

Samasthiti   Ekam   Dve   Trini   Catvari   Panca   Sat   Sapta   Astau   Nava

Dasa   Ekadasa   Dvadasa   Trayodasa   Caturdasa   Pancadasa   Sodasa   Saptadasa   Samasthiti

## STANDING SEQUENCE

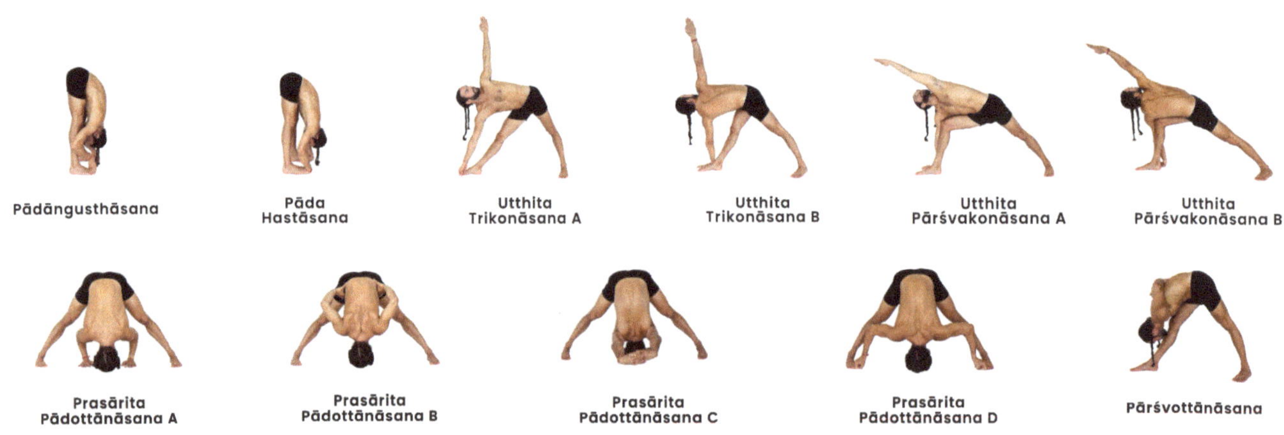

Pādāngusthāsana   Pāda Hastāsana   Utthita Trikonāsana A   Utthita Trikonāsana B   Utthita Pārśvakonāsana A   Utthita Pārśvakonāsana B

Prasārita Pādottānāsana A   Prasārita Pādottānāsana B   Prasārita Pādottānāsana C   Prasārita Pādottānāsana D   Pārśvottānāsana

**ASHTANGA YOGA** SECOND SERIES
BY ROSS STAMBAUGH • KPJAYI AUTHORIZED LEVEL 2

# SEATED SEQUENCE

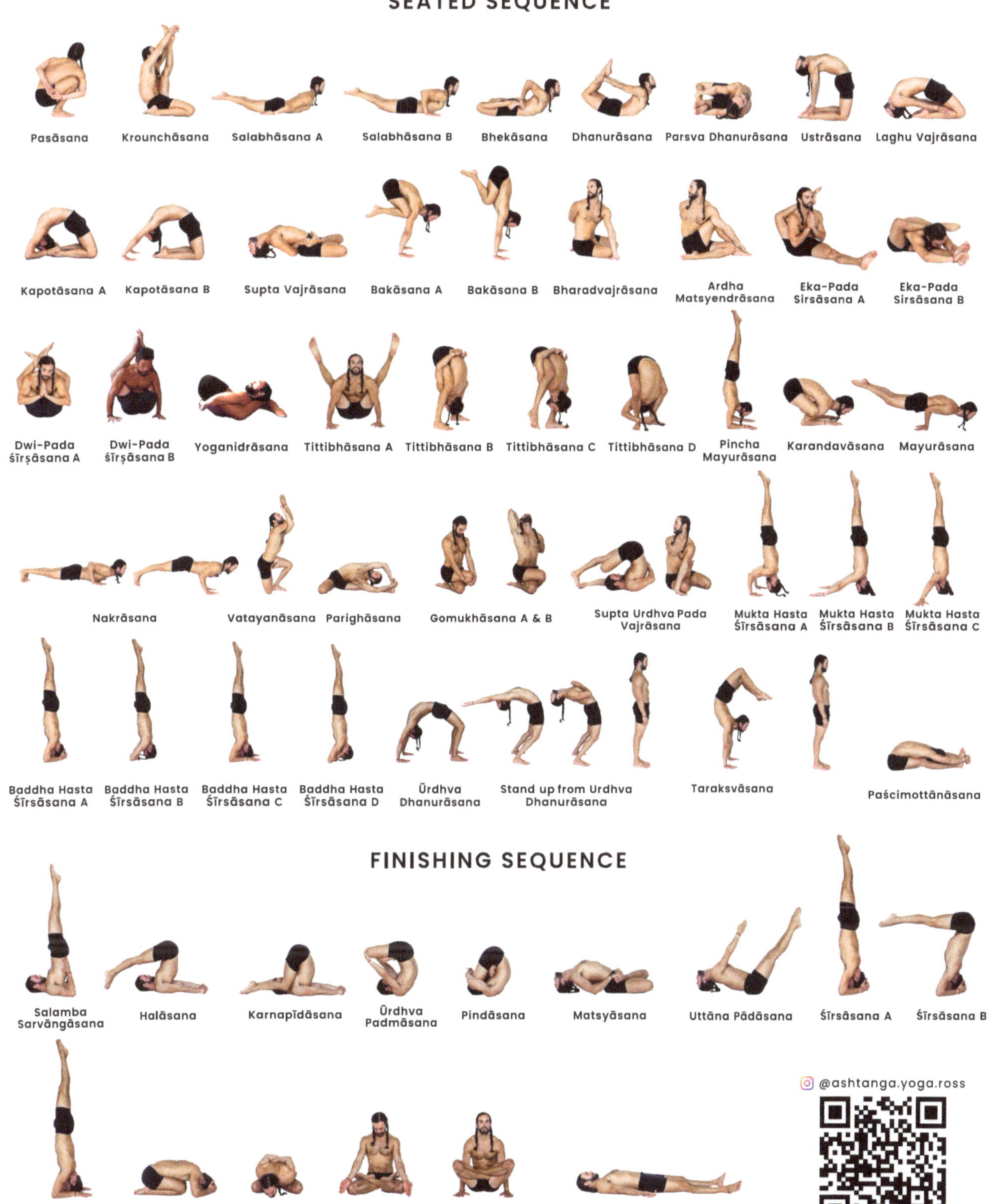

Pasāsana · Krounchāsana · Salabhāsana A · Salabhāsana B · Bhekāsana · Dhanurāsana · Parsva Dhanurāsana · Ustrāsana · Laghu Vajrāsana

Kapotāsana A · Kapotāsana B · Supta Vajrāsana · Bakāsana A · Bakāsana B · Bharadvajrāsana · Ardha Matsyendrāsana · Eka-Pada Sirsāsana A · Eka-Pada Sirsāsana B

Dwi-Pada Śīrṣāsana A · Dwi-Pada Śīrṣāsana B · Yoganidrāsana · Tittibhāsana A · Tittibhāsana B · Tittibhāsana C · Tittibhāsana D · Pincha Mayurāsana · Karandavāsana · Mayurāsana

Nakrāsana · Vatayanāsana · Parighāsana · Gomukhāsana A & B · Supta Urdhva Pada Vajrāsana · Mukta Hasta Śīrṣāsana A · Mukta Hasta Śīrṣāsana B · Mukta Hasta Śīrṣāsana C

Baddha Hasta Śīrṣāsana A · Baddha Hasta Śīrṣāsana B · Baddha Hasta Śīrṣāsana C · Baddha Hasta Śīrṣāsana D · Ūrdhva Dhanurāsana · Stand up from Urdhva Dhanurāsana · Taraksvāsana · Paścimottānāsana

# FINISHING SEQUENCE

Salamba Sarvāngāsana · Halāsana · Karnapīdāsana · Ūrdhva Padmāsana · Pindāsana · Matsyāsana · Uttāna Pādāsana · Śīrsāsana A · Śīrsāsana B

Śīrsāsana C · Rest · Yogamudra · Padmāsana · Utpluthih · Take Rest



**ASHTANGA YOGA** SECOND SERIES
BY ROSS STAMBAUGH • KPJAYI AUTHORIZED LEVEL 2

# Temples of Gokulum, Mysore India
## by: Sat Inder Kalasa @in_her_lap

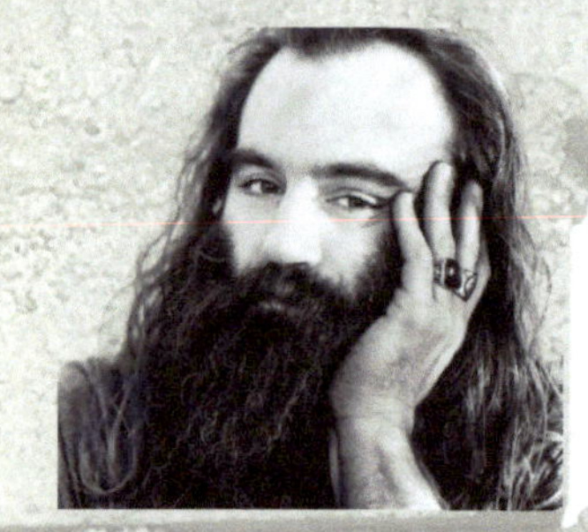

Temple Tours around Mysore with Sat Inder:     My first trip to Mysore I was really drawn to the temples, this was early 2014.  I've always been interested in an alternative spiritual or religious experience to the one I was brought up in.  But that trip I only went into the well known Ganesha temple in Gokulam because I was nervous with not knowing what to do. I quickly discovered that they were happy to tell me what the rituals were and how to partake in them.  And on subsequent trips I learned from Indian friends about other temples, and the priests in each one would show me what to do.  Until about 2016 when other yoga students saw me either coming out of temples, or going into them and began asking me to show them what to do, where temples were and they offered to pay me.  So I checked in with the priests at several temples and they all encouraged me to teach people what I knew so they could also benefit from the temple energy.  And so I did, but only a couple times that year.  In 2017 is when I really began to discover some links to temples and building specific types of tours to give people insights into the differences and similarities within all of them they would see around town. Saturday to visit Hanuman and Shani Deva, plus a few others. Friday nights to visit several Devi temples.

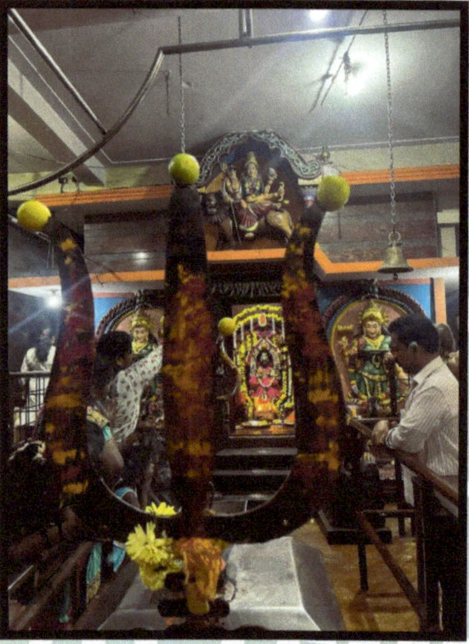

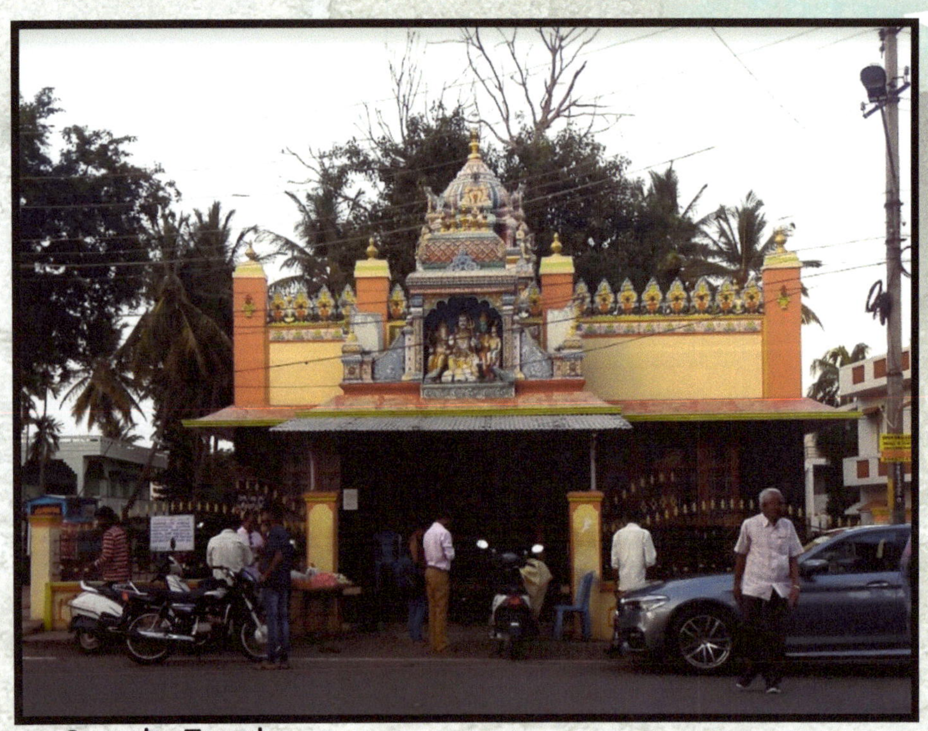

Ganesha Temple

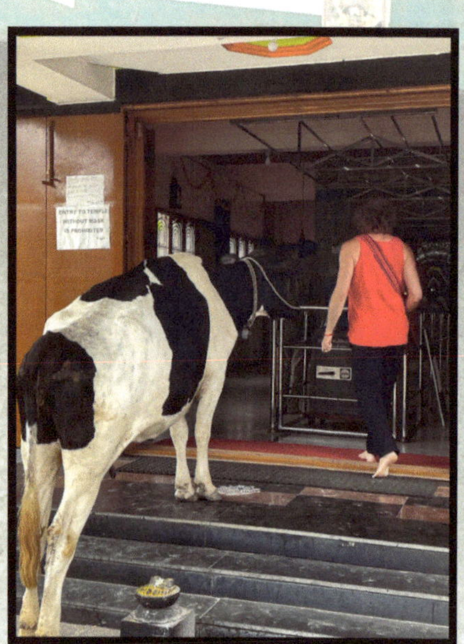

Mondays driving to Nanjangud or around Mysore to different Shiva temples. I'd meet the people early and explain the rituals, tell them about the different Gods being worshipped on different days and answer any questions they had before, and during the tour. We ride around in rickshaws or on scooters, or my Saturday tour is walking for those interested in that. I only charge 500 rupees which is about $6 and very affordable for most foreigners, but sometimes Indians come too who want to reconnect with their culture and can't afford that much, and I have them come anyway. It is a small income for me and helps in my time in India but is more about sharing this lovely culture that has welcomed me fully and come to be my home...

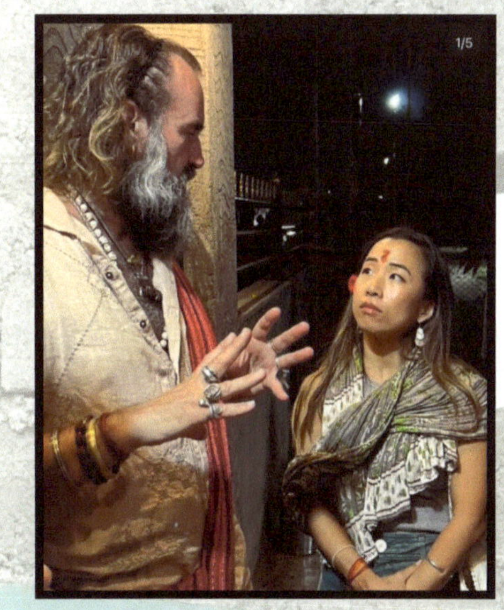

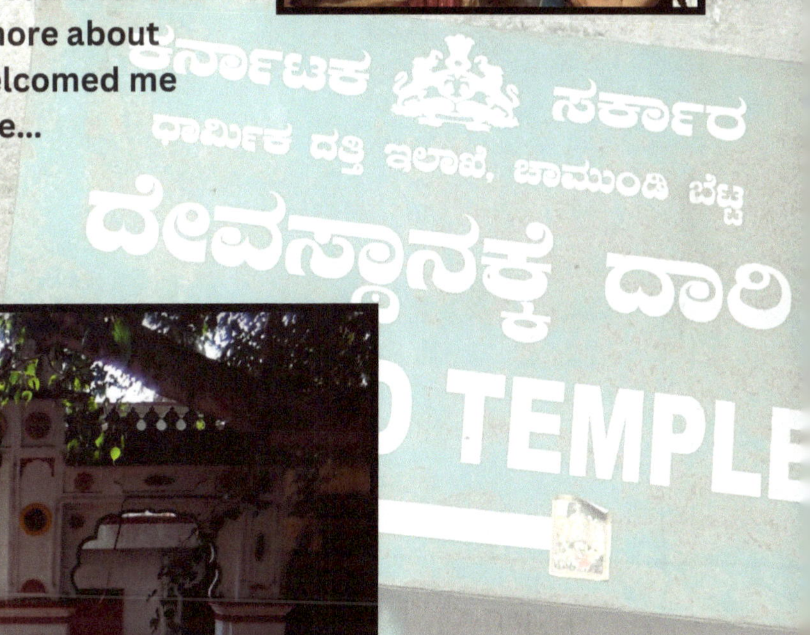

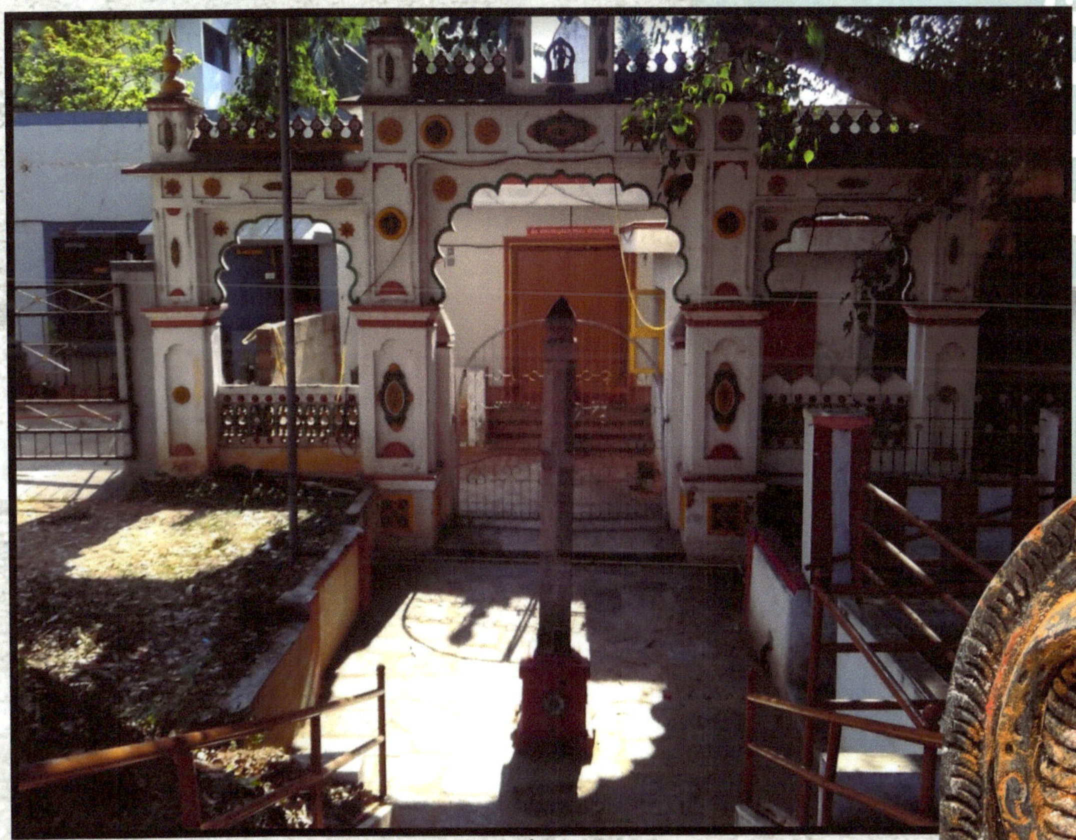

Sri Balasubramaya Swamy Temple

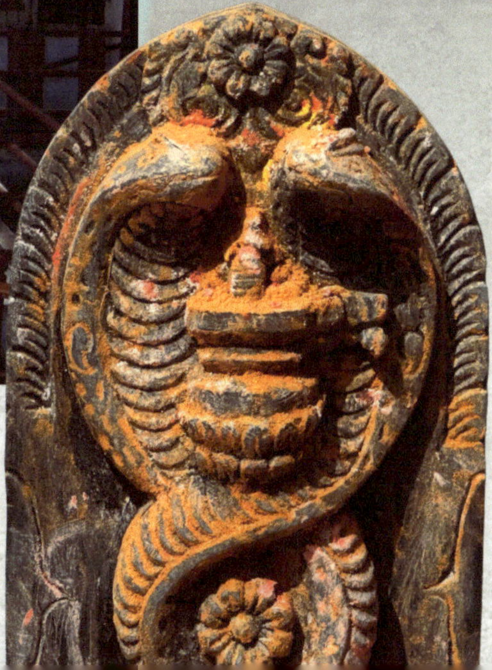

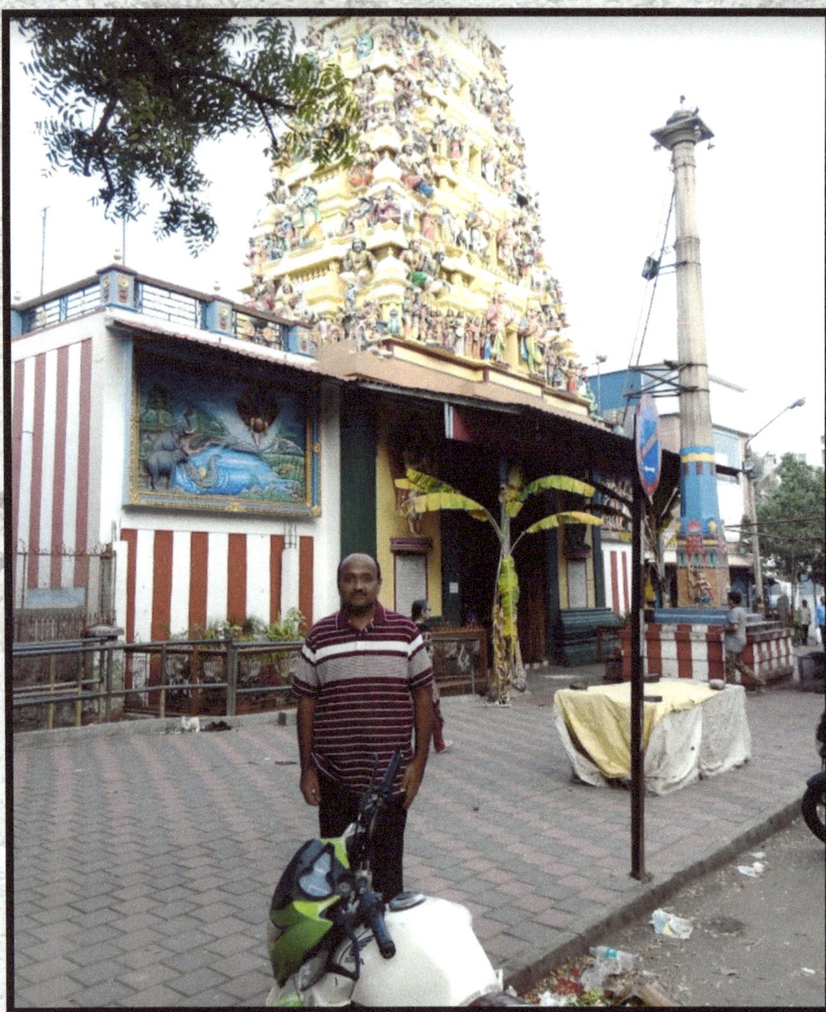

Sri Venkateswara Temple Mysore

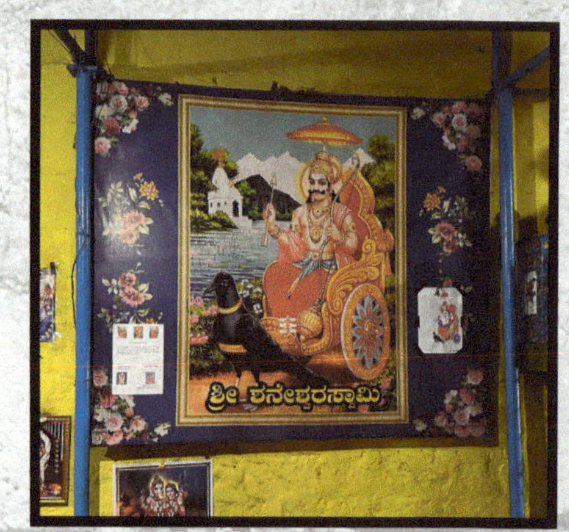



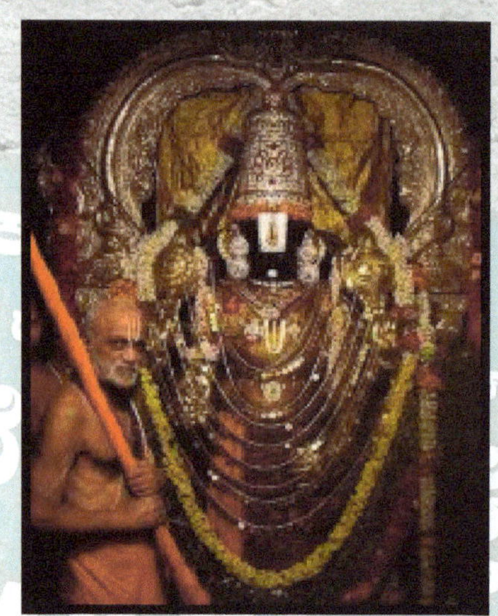



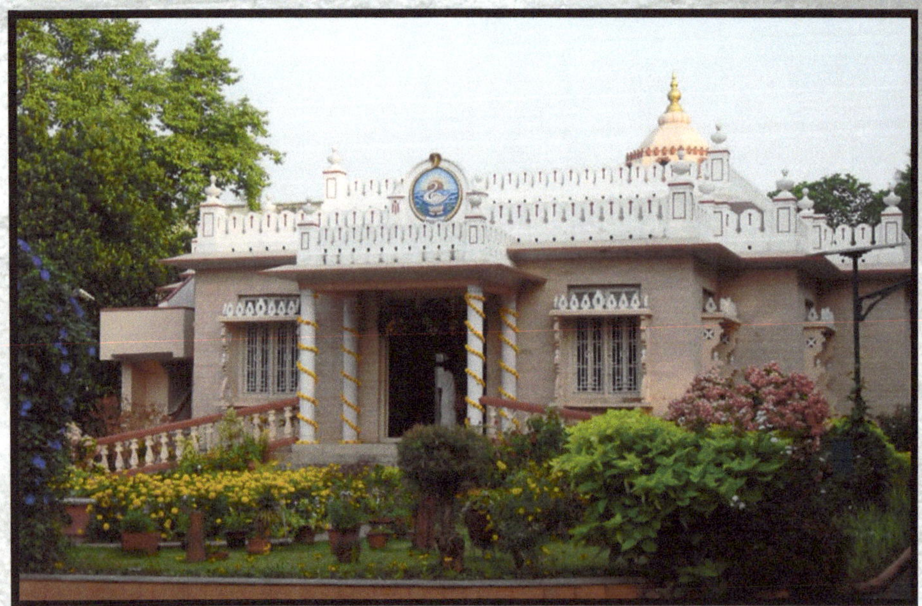

Sri Ramakrishna Temple

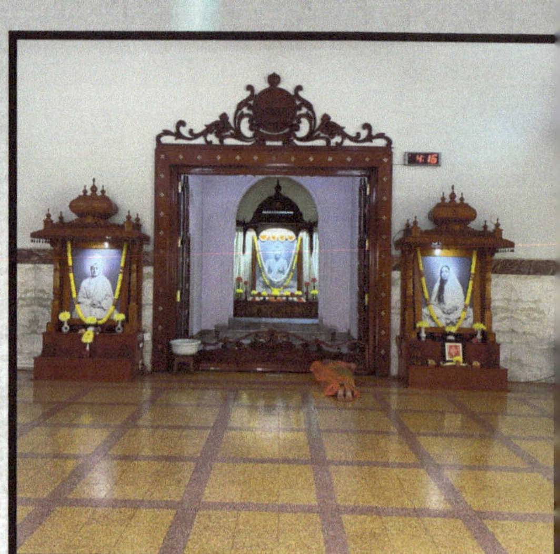

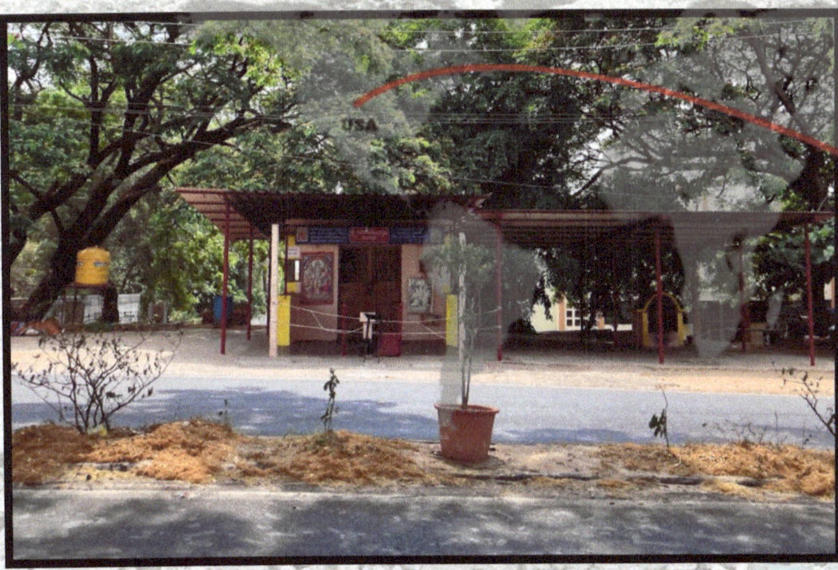

Sri Veeranjaneya Swamy Temple

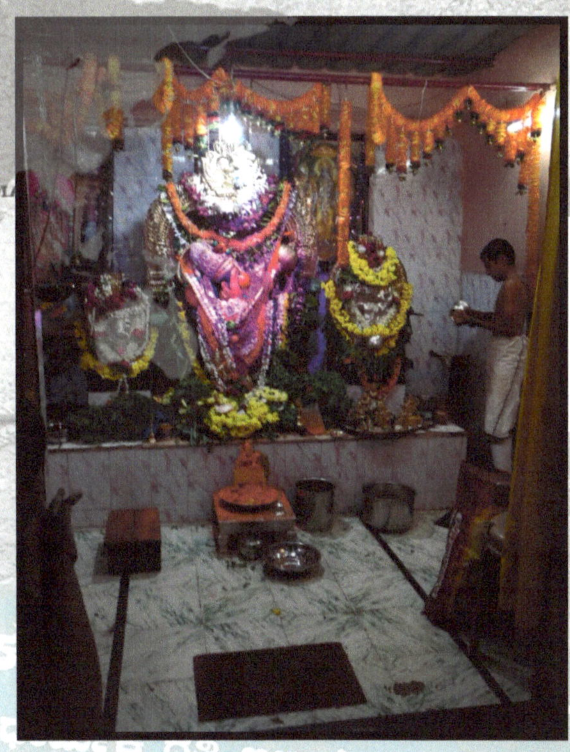

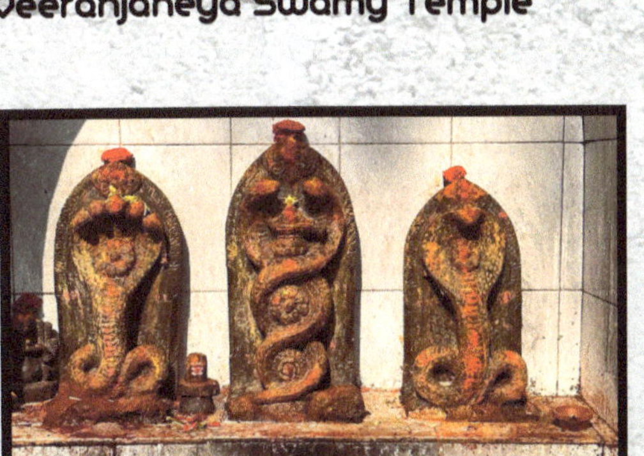

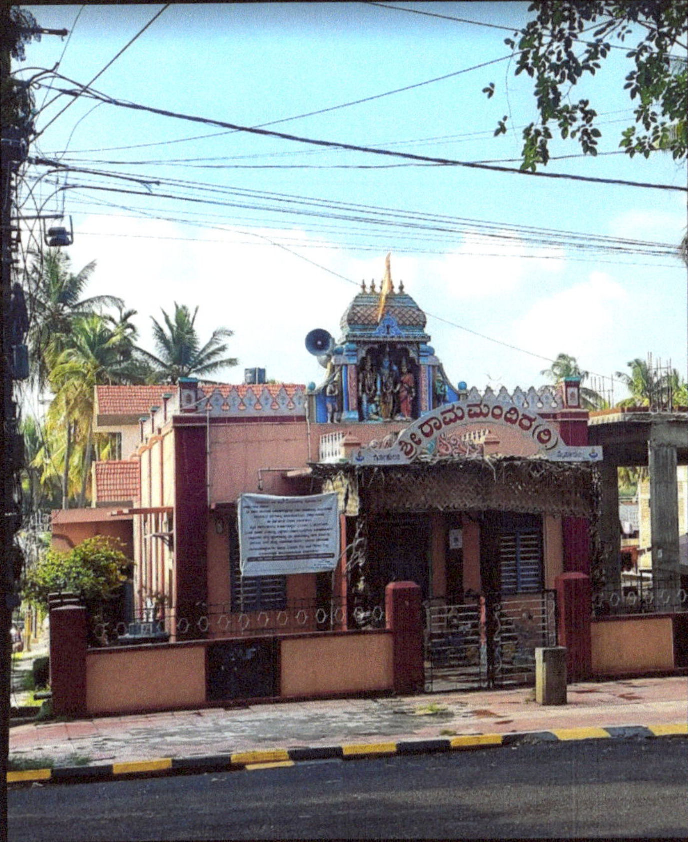

Rama Mandira

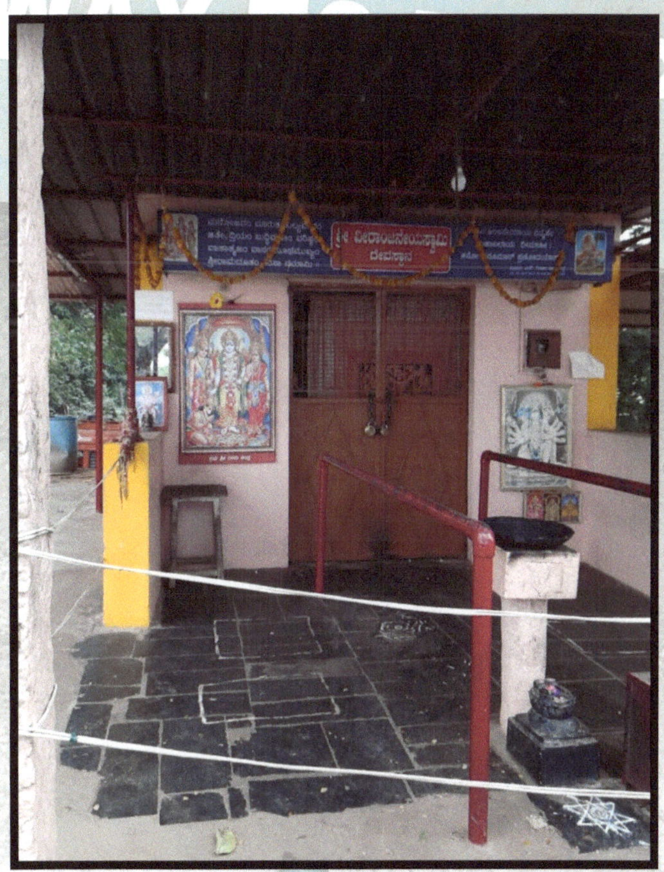

# Things to consider while visiting a temple.

Visiting a Hindu temple is a spiritual and cultural experience, and there are certain protocols and etiquette to follow to show respect to the deity and the sacred space. While specific customs and practices may vary based on the temple's traditions and regional customs, here are some general guidelines:

1. **Dress Code:** Modest attire is typically expected when visiting a Hindu temple. Avoid wearing revealing clothing, shorts, or sleeveless tops. It's common for visitors to remove their shoes before entering the temple, so wearing footwear that is easy to slip on and off is recommended.

2. **Purification:** Before entering the inner sanctum of the temple or approaching the deity, it's customary to wash your hands and feet if facilities are available. Some temples may provide a water tank or basin for this purpose.

3. **Respectful Behavior:** Maintain a quiet and respectful demeanor inside the temple. Avoid talking loudly, using mobile phones, or engaging in disruptive behavior. Photography may be prohibited or restricted in certain areas, so it's best to ask for permission before taking pictures.

4. **Offerings:** It's common to bring offerings such as flowers, fruits, sweets, or incense when visiting a temple. These offerings are usually placed before the deity as a symbol of devotion. If you're unsure about the appropriate offerings, you can ask the temple staff or priests for guidance.

5. **Observing Rituals:** Observe and respect the rituals and customs taking place in the temple. If a priest is performing prayers or rituals, it's customary to wait quietly until they are finished before approaching the deity.

6. **Circumambulation:** In some temples, devotees perform circumambulation (pradakshina) around the inner sanctum or the main deity. This involves walking clockwise around the shrine as a form of reverence. Follow the direction of the flow and be mindful of other worshippers.

7. **Prostrations and Prayers:** If you wish to offer prayers or make prostrations before the deity, it's important to do so with sincerity and reverence. Bow respectfully and offer your prayers silently or aloud, depending on your preference.

8. **Respect for Sacred Objects:** Avoid touching or pointing your feet towards sacred objects, idols, or images of the deity. Feet are considered impure in Hindu culture, so it's respectful to keep them pointed away from anything sacred.

9. **Follow Temple Rules:** Each temple may have specific rules and regulations for visitors. Pay attention to signs and instructions provided by the temple authorities, and abide by any guidelines they have in place.

By following these protocols and showing respect for the traditions of the temple, you can have a meaningful and respectful experience during your visit. If you're unsure about any customs or practices, don't hesitate to ask the temple staff or fellow worshippers for guidance.

From the Brihadaranyaka Upanishad, this
mantra means:

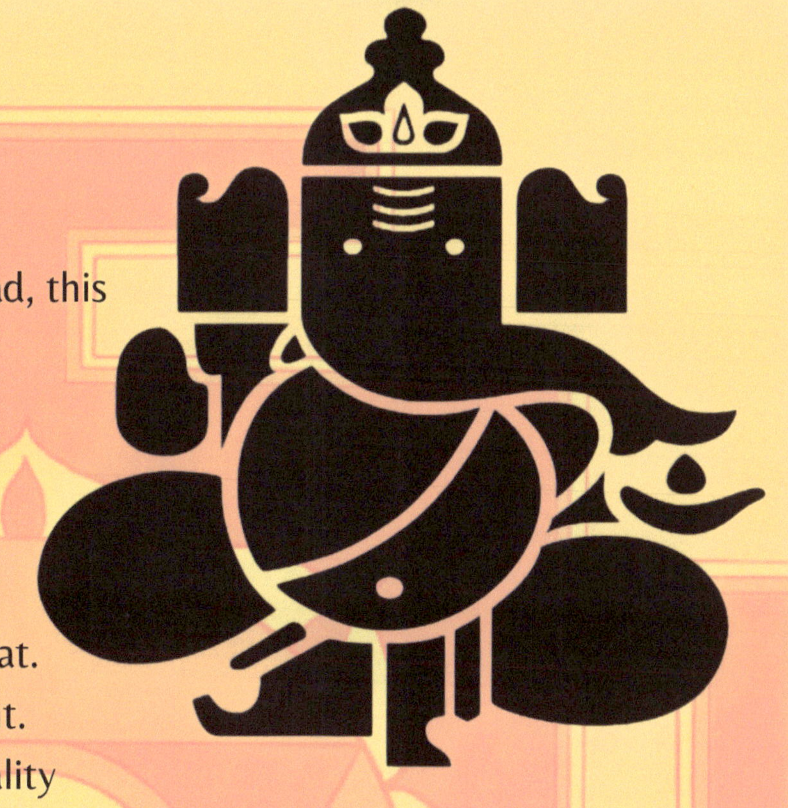

ॐ असतो मा सद्गमय ।
तमसो मा ज्योतिर्गमय ।
मृत्योर्मा अमृतं गमय ।
ॐ शान्तिः शान्तिः शान्तिः ॥

Lead me from the asat to the sat.
Lead me from darkness to light.
Lead me from death to immortality
Om Peace Peace Peace.

# om asato mā sad gamaya

# tamaso mā jyotir gamaya

# mrtyor mā amrtaṁ gamaya

# oṁ śāntiḥ, śāntiḥ, śāntiḥ

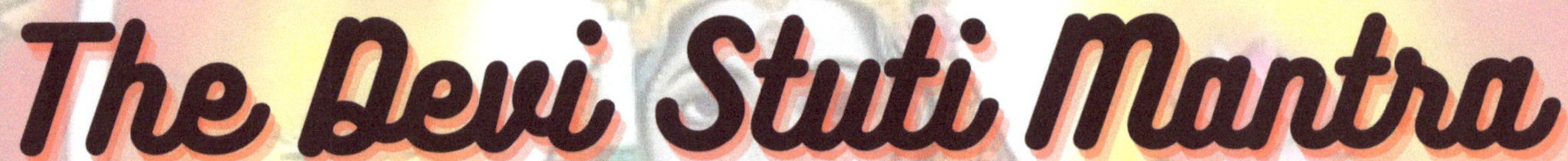

# The Devi Stuti Mantra

॥ या देवी सर्वभुतेषु शक्तिरूपेण संस्थिता

या देवी सर्वभुतेषु शक्तिरूपेण संस्थिता

या देवी सर्वभुतेषु मातृरूपेण संस्थिता

या देवी सर्वभुतेषु बुद्धिरूपेण संस्थिता

नमस्तस्यै नमस्तस्यै नमस्तस्यै नमो नमः ॥

YA DEVI SARVA BHUTESHU, SHANTI RUPENA SANGSTHITA

YA DEVI SARVA BHUTESHU, SHAKTI RUPENA SANGSTHITA

YA DEVI SARVA BHUTESHU, MATRI RUPENA SANGSTHITA

YAA DEVI SARVA BHUTESHU, BUDDHI RUPENA SANGSTHITA

NAMASTASYAI, NAMASTASYAI, NAMASTASYAI, NAMO NAMAHA

MEANING – THE GODDESS WHO IS OMNIPRESENT AS THE
PERSONIFICATION OF THE UNIVERSAL MOTHER
THE GODDESS WHO IS OMNIPRESENT AS THE EMBODIMENT OF THE
POWER
THE GODDESS WHO IS OMNIPRESENT AS THE SYMBOL OF PEACE
OH, GODDESS (DEVI) WHO RESIDES EVERYWHERE IN ALL LIVING
BEINGS AS INTELLIGENCE AND BEAUTY,
I BOW TO HER, I BOW TO HER, I BOW TO HER AGAIN & AGAIN.

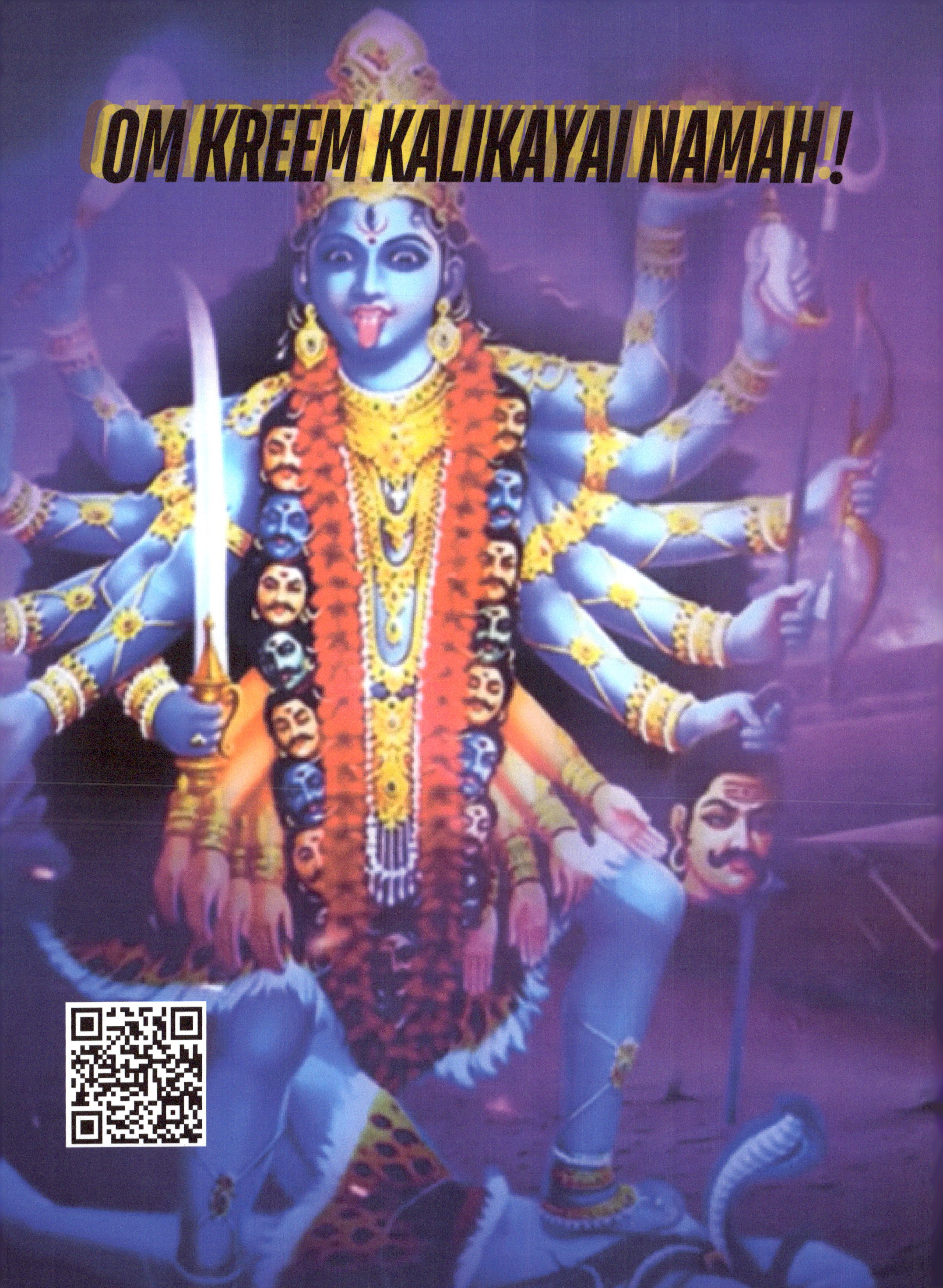

OM KREEM KALIKAYAI NAMAH!

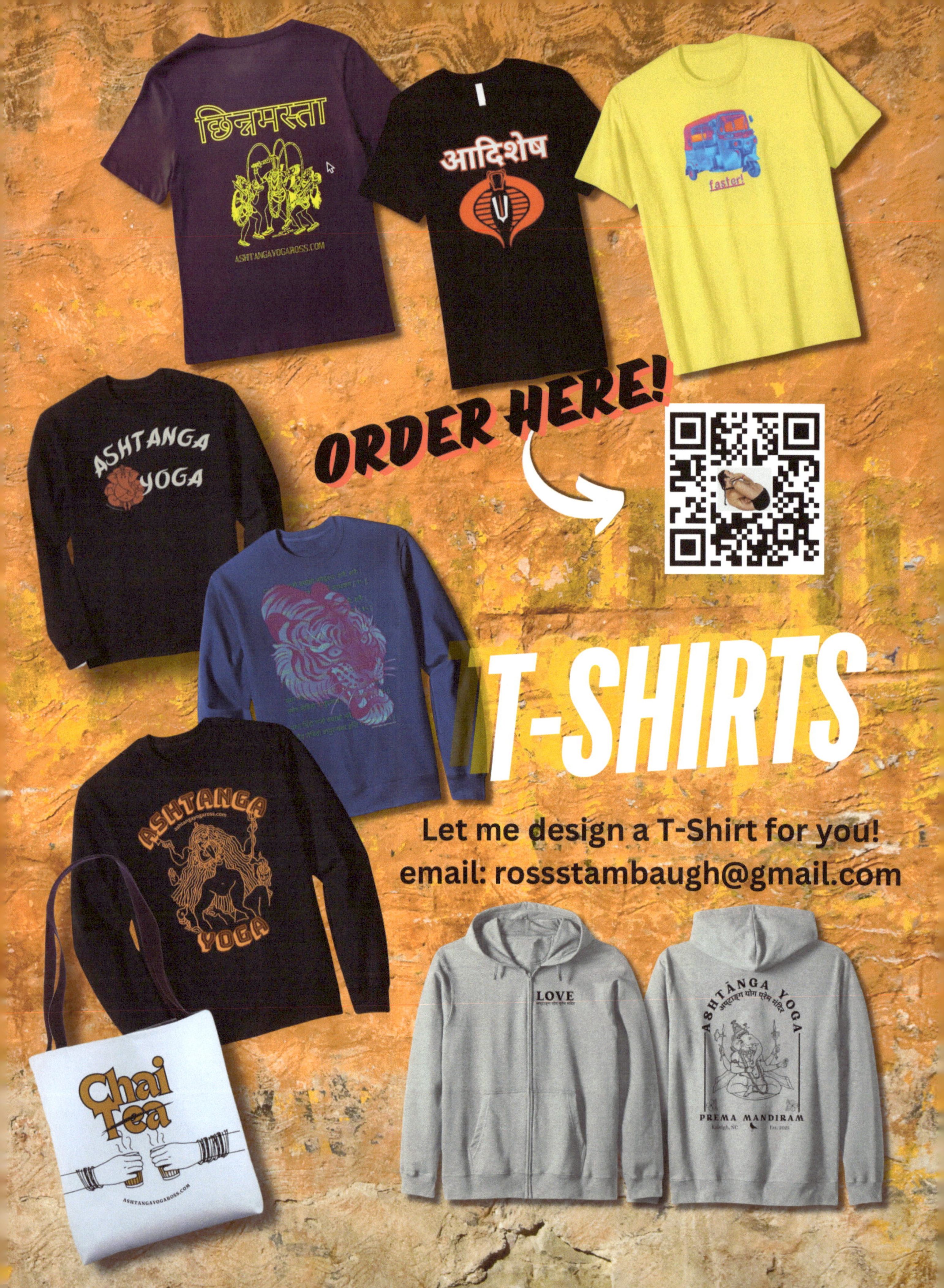
छिन्नमस्ता
ASHTANGAYOGAROSS.COM
आदिशेष
faster!
ASHTANGA YOGA
ASHTANGA YOGA
ashtangayogaross.com
Chai Tea
ASHTANGAYOGAROSS.COM
ORDER HERE!
T-SHIRTS
Let me design a T-Shirt for you!
email: rossstambaugh@gmail.com
LOVE
ASHTANGA YOGA
PREMA MANDIRAM
Raleigh, NC    Est. 2023

तदा द्रष्टुः स्वरूपेऽवस्थानम् ॥३॥
ĀTMAN 1
Private Yoga Magazine
ashtangayogaross.com
Shani Dev Publishing

तदा द्रष्टुः स्वरूपेऽवस्थानम् ॥३॥
ĀTMAN 2
Private Yoga Magazine
Shani Dev Publishing
तदा द्रष्टुः स्वरूपेऽवस्थानम् ॥३॥
ĀTMAN 3
Private Yoga Magazine
Shani Dev Publishing
तदा द्रष्टुः स्वरूपेऽवस्थानम् ॥३॥
ĀTMAN 4
Private Yoga Magazine
ashtangayogaross.com
Shani Dev Publishing

# BOOKS!!!

ASHTĀNGA
YOGA
Counted Primary Series
Ross Stambaugh

ASHTĀNGA
YOGA
Counted Second Series
by Ross Stambaugh

Ashtanga Svādhyāya
Self-Study Guide

Ross Stambaugh

The Yoga Sutras Flipbook

Ross Stambaugh

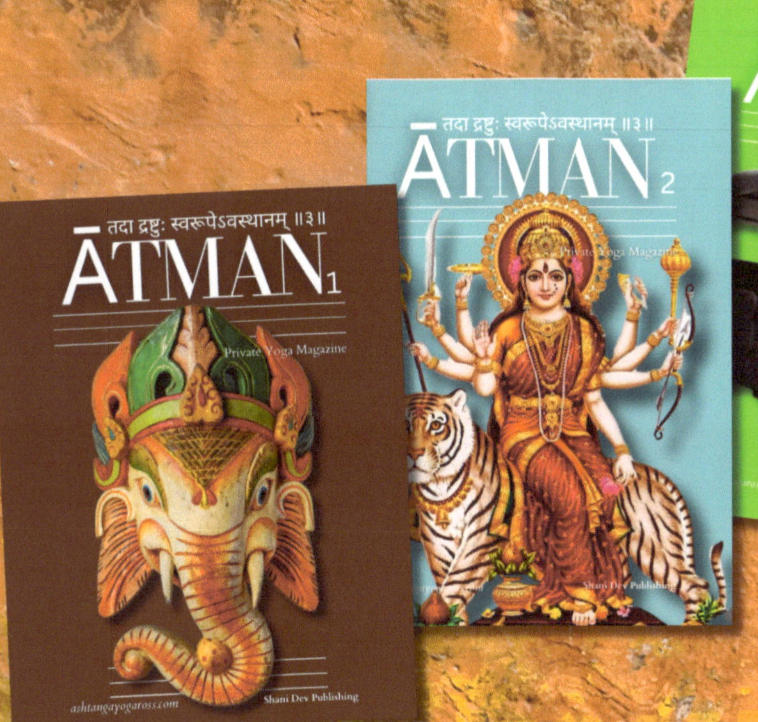

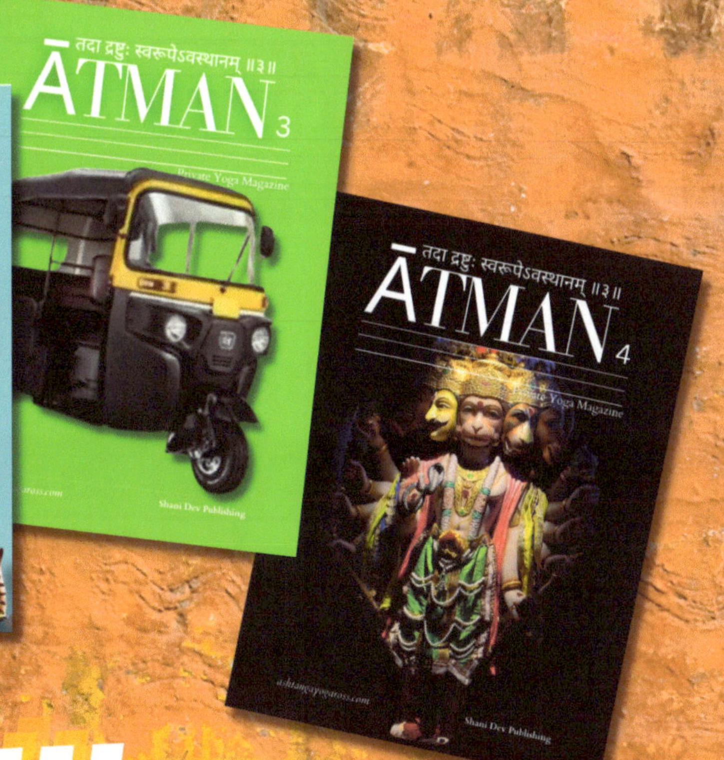

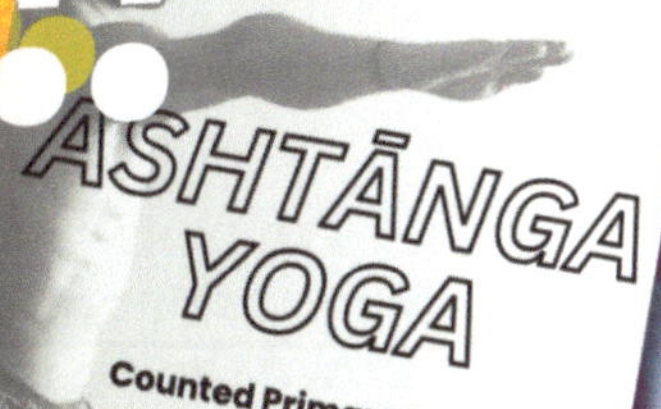

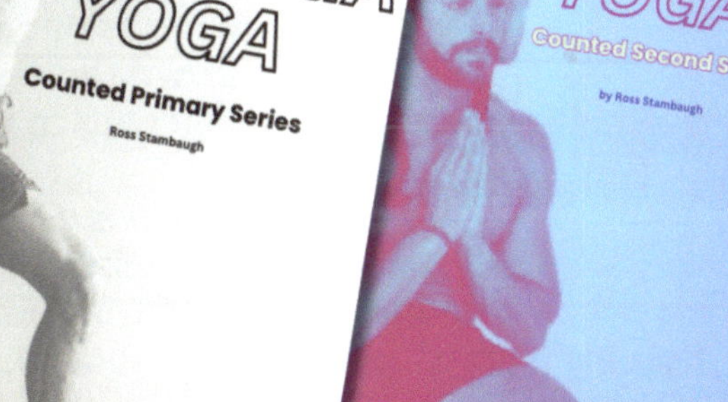

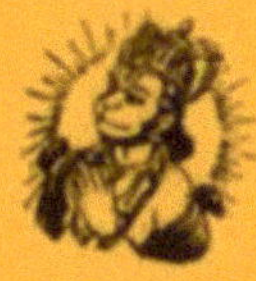

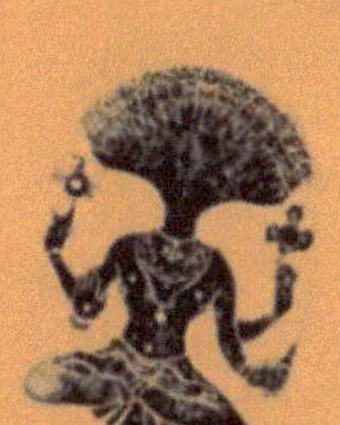

# Om
# Vande Gurunam Charanaravinde
# Sandarshita Svatma Sukava
# Bodhe
# Nih Sreyase Jangalikayamane
# Samsara Halahala Mohashantyai
# Abahu Purushakaram
# Shankhacakrsi Dharinam
# Sahasra Sirasam Svetam
# Pranamami Patanjalim
# Om

I bow to the lotus feet of the Supreme Guru
which awaken insight into the happiness of pure Being,
which are the refuge, the jungle physician,
which eliminate the delusion caused by the poisonous herb of Samsara (conditioned
existence).
I prostrate before the sage Patanjali
who has thousands of radiant, white heads (as the divine serpent, Ananta)
and who has, as far as his arms, assumed the form of a man
holding a conch shell (divine sound), a wheel (discus of light or infinite time) and a
sword (discrimination).
om

# Om
# Svasthi Praja Bhyaha Pari Pala Yantam
# Nya Yena Margena Mahim Mahishaha
# Go Brahmanebhyaha Shubamastu
# Nityam
# Lokah Samastah Sukhino Bhavantu
# Om Shanti Shanti Shantihi

May the rulers of the earth keep to the path of virtue
For protecting the welfare of all generations.
May the religious, and all peoples be forever blessed,
May all beings everywhere be happy and free
Om peace, peace, perfect peace

Originally found in the Krishna Yajurveda Taittiriya Upanishad (2.2.2), it is often chanted at the start of a school class or at the beginning of a yoga practice.

# om saha nā vavatu

# saha nau bhunaktu

# saha vīryam karavāvahai

# tejasvināvadhītamastu

# mā vidviṣāvahai

# om śāntiḥ śāntiḥ śāntiḥ

1: Om, Together may we two Move (in our Studies, the Teacher and the Student),
2: Together may we two Relish (our Studies, the Teacher and the Student),
3: Together may we perform (our Studies) with Vigour(with deep Concentration),
4: May what has been Studied by us be filled with the Brilliance (of Understanding, leading to Knowledge); May it Not give rise to Hostility (due to lack of Understanding),
5: Om Peace, Peace, Peace.

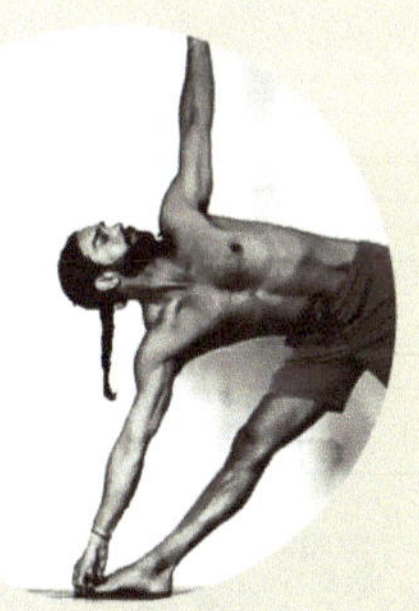

### Foundations

The first 11 asanas of the Primary Series will be introduced. Modifications and assists will be shown. Students will have an understanding how to start an Ashtanga Practice at home or in a yoga shala.

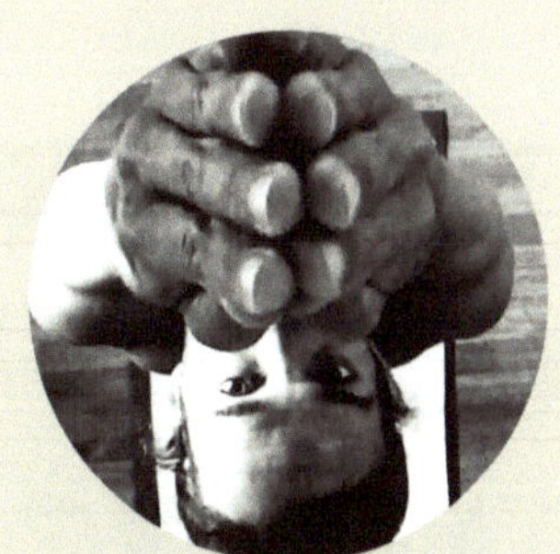

### Mysore Style

Students will be taught the Ashtanga Yoga method as it is still taught in Mysore, India today. Students will practice their asanas and receive 1-on-1 instruction, assists, and modifications in a group setting.

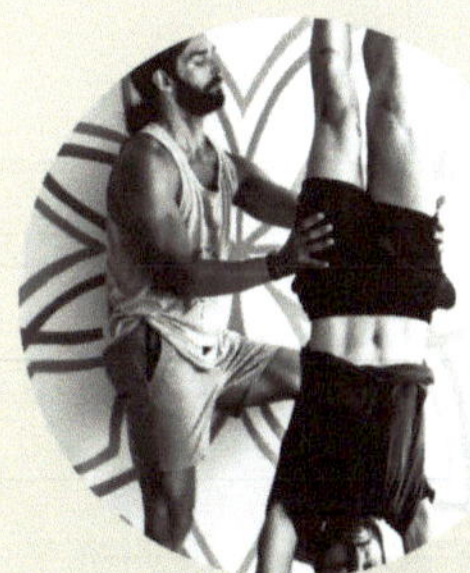

### Hidden Handstands

This workshop is for handstand lovers or those that wish to develop a handstand into their daily yoga practice. Mix of drills and skills is the main focus. Students should feel comfortable completing Sun Salutations and should be practicing yoga on a regular basis.

# ashtangayogaross.com

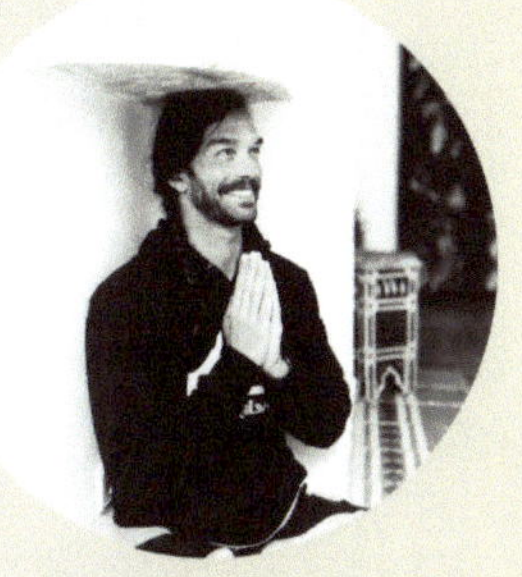

### Sutra Studies

This workshop will focus on the Yoga Sutras of Patanjali. Students will look at different translations of this philosophical text and engage in a meaningful conversation. Guidebook provided.

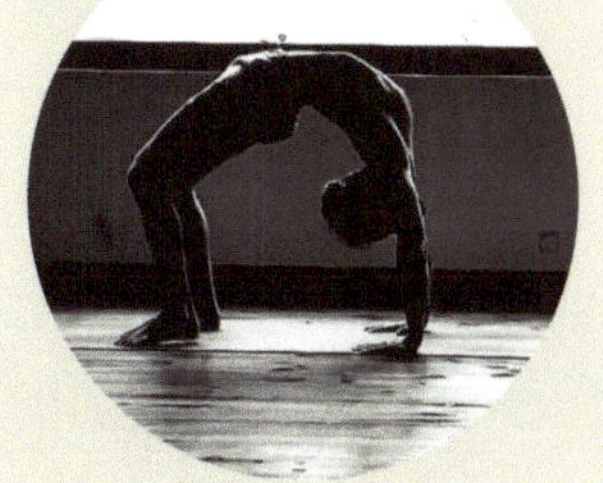

### Better Backbends

This workshop will look at backbends from the Ashtanga Primary & Secondary series. Theory will be discussed, followed by practice, ways to modify, change and assist. *Students should be comfortable pressing into "wheel pose" is required.

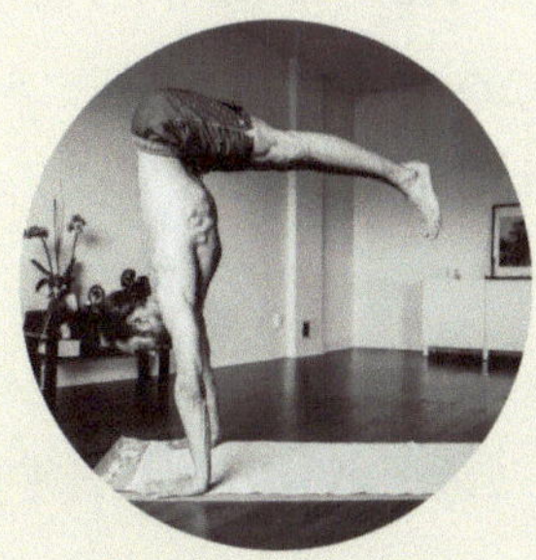

### Arm Balances & Inversions

If you enjoy being upside down or looking to improve your arm balancing skills, then learn new techniques combined with strength. The focus is developing proprioceptive skills (how you move and maintain position in time and space) with focus and balance.

# WORKSHOPS THAT I OFFER

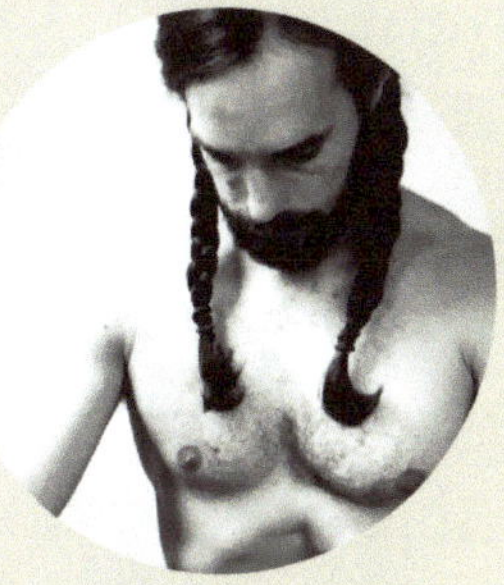

### Pranayama - Breath of Yoga

Are you ready to bridge the gap between asana and starting an independent pranayama (yogic breathing) practice? Theory will be discussed, followed by the 6 traditional pranayama techniques, chanting, anatomical alignment, and more.

# #YOGIS HELPING YOGIS

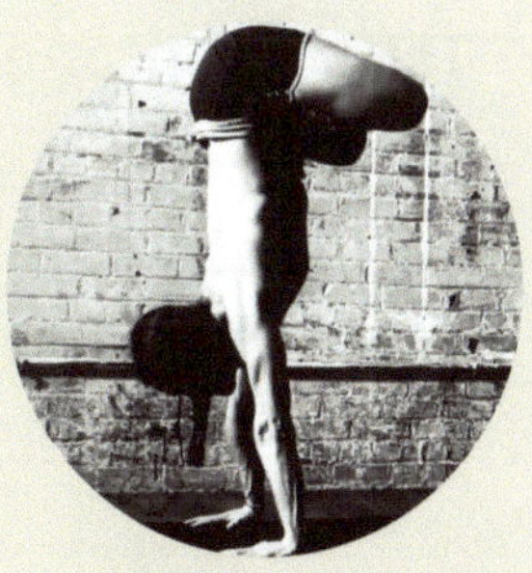

### Yogis Helping Yogis

This workshop is for yoga teachers or for students aiming to start teaching. This workshop will cover how manage a room with students of various skill levels, understand proper etiquette, how and when to use props, hands-on assists, and the complexities of running an Ashtanga centered class.

# ***WHY ARE HINDU GODS SHOWN HAVING MULTIPLE ARMS?***

In Sanatan Dharma, Deities are often depicted with multiple arms. These many arms become visible when they are battling with cosmic forces. The multiple arms of Hindu Gods and Goddesses show the greater power of Deities over humans.

According to the science of Hindu iconography there are three categories of icons.

- Santa(peaceful) - icons in this category have only 2 or 4 arms.
- Vira(hero) - icons in this category can have 2 or 4 or 6 arms and are usually depicted in confrontational posture.
- Ugra(wrathful) - icons with 6 or more arms in full battle engagement.

Most Hindu deities are depicted with four arms, these represent:

- The cardinal directions: indicating that the god is all pervading and has perfect dominion over all the directions.
- The four divisions of society: intellectuals, administrators, entrepreneurs, and workers.
- The four stages of life: student, householder, retirement and renunciate.
- The four aspects of Hindu psychology: the lower cogitative mind (manas) the intellect (buddhi), ego (ahamkara) and consciousness (cit).
- The four levels of consciousness: waking (jagrata), dream (svapna), sub-consciousness (susupti) and transcendental consciousness (turiya).
- The four essential components of dharma: truth (satya), meditation (tapa), compassion (daya), and charity (dãna).

- The four aims of human endeavor (purusarthas): pleasure (kama), prosperity (artha), righteousness (dharma) and liberation (moksa).
- The four "immeasurable" qualities:
- friendliness (maitri), compassion (karuna), empathetic joy (mudita) and non-attachment (upeksa).
- The four Vedic fires: havaniya, garhapatya, avasthay and sabhya.
- The four stages of Liberation: salokya, samipya, sãrupya and sayujya
- The four types of Yogas: jhana(wisdom), bhakti(devotion), karma(actions) and saranägati(surrender).
- The four qualities of all manifested beings: category (jäti), attributes (guna), function (kriya) and relationship (sambandha).
- Some icons are depicted as having 8 arms. This also represents the complete dominion over all the directions, as well as the eight divine preserving powers (sakti) which are:
- Health (arogya)
- Knowledge (jñana)
- Wealth (dhana)
- Organization (sampadanam)
- Cooperation (sahodyogah)
- Fame (kirti)
- Courage (dhrti), and
- Truth (satyam)